Genitourinary Ultrasound II

Guest Editors

PAUL S. SIDHU, MBBS, MRCP, FRCR
MUKUND JOSHI, MD

ULTRASOUND CLINICS

www.ultrasound.theclinics.com

Consulting Editor
VIKRAM DOGRA, MD

October 2010 • Volume 5 • Number 4

SAUNDERS an imprint of ELSEVIER, Inc.

W.B. SAUNDERS COMPANY
A Division of Elsevier Inc.

1600 John F. Kennedy Boulevard ● Suite 1800 ● Philadelphia, Pennsylvania 19103-2899

http://www.theclinics.com

ULTRASOUND CLINICS Volume 5, Number 4
October 2010 ISSN 1556-858X, ISBN-13: 978-1-4557-0405-7

Editor: Barton Dudlick

Ultrasound Clinics (ISSN 1556-858X) is published quarterly by W.B. Saunders, 360 Park Avenue South, New York, NY 10010-1710. Months of publication are January, April, July, and October. Business and editorial offices: 1600 John F. Kennedy Boulevard, Suite 1800, Philadelphia, Pennsylvania 19103-2899. Accounting and circulation offices: 6277 Sea Harbor Drive, Orlando, FL 32887-4800. Periodicals postage paid at New York, NY, and additional mailing offices. Subscription prices are $225 per year for (US individuals), $279 per year for (US institutions), $107 per year for (US students and residents), $253 per year for (Canadian individuals), $312 per year for (Canadian institutions), $269 per year for (international individuals), $312 per year for (international institutions), and $129 per year for (Canadian and foreign students/residents). To receive student/resident rate, orders must be accompanied by name of affiliated institution, date of term, and the signature of program/residency coordinator on institution letterhead. Orders will be billed at individual rate until proof of status is received. Foreign air speed delivery is included in all Clinics subscription prices. All prices are subject to change without notice. **POSTMASTER:** Send address changes to *Ultrasound Clinics,* Elsevier Health Sciences Division, Subscription Customer Service, 3251 Riverport Lane, Maryland Heights, MO 63043. **Customer Service (orders, claims, online, change of address): Telephone: 1-800-654-2452 (U.S. and Canada); 314-447-8871 (outside U.S. and Canada). Fax: 314-447-8029. E-mail: journalscustomerservice-usa@elsevier.com (for print support); journalsonlinesupport-usa@elsevier.com (for online support).**

Reprints: For copies of 100 or more, of articles in this publication, please contact the Commercial Reprints Department, Elsevier Inc., 360 Park Avenue South, New York, NY 10010-1710. Tel.: (+1) 212-633-3812; Fax: (+1) 212-462-1935; E-mail: reprints@elsevier.com.

Printed and bound by CPI Group (UK) Ltd, Croydon, CR0 4YY
Transferred to Digital Print 2012

Contributors

CONSULTING EDITOR

VIKRAM S. DOGRA, MD
Professor of Radiology, Urology, and
Biomedical Engineering, Director of Ultrasound
and Associate Chair for Education and
Research, Department of Imaging Sciences,
University of Rochester School of Medicine
and Dentistry, Rochester, New York

GUEST EDITORS

PAUL S. SIDHU, MBBS, MRCP, FRCR
Consultant Radiologist and Senior Lecturer,
Department of Diagnostic Radiology, King's
College Hospital, Denmark Hill, London, United
Kingdom

MUKUND JOSHI, MD
Dr Joshi's Imaging Clinic, Mumbai,
Maharashtra, India

AUTHORS

SHWETA BHATT, MD
Assistant Professor, Department of Radiology,
University of Rochester Medical Center,
Rochester, New York

VIKRAM S. DOGRA, MD
Professor of Radiology, Urology, and
Biomedical Engineering, Director of Ultrasound
and Associate Chair for Education and
Research, Department of Imaging Sciences,
University of Rochester School of Medicine
and Dentistry, Rochester, New York

CHRIS J. HARVEY, MBBS, MRCP, FRCR
Consultant Radiologist, Department of
Imaging, Hammersmith Hospital, London,
United Kingdom

ERKAN KISMALI, MD
Staff Radiologist, Department of Radiology,
University of Ege, School of Medicine, Izmir,
Turkey

ASHWIN LAWANDE, DNB
Dr Joshi's Imaging Clinic, Mumbai,
Maharashtra, India

PHILLIP FC. LUNG, MRCS, FRCR
Specialist Registrar in Radiology, Department
of Radiology, King's College Hospital, London,
United Kingdom

PAUL S. SIDHU, MBBS, MRCP, FRCR
Consultant Radiologist, Department of
Radiology, King's College Hospital, London,
United Kingdom

RAVINDER SIDHU, MD
Assistant Professor, Department of Radiology,
University of Rochester Medical Center,
Rochester, New York

AHMET T. TURGUT, MD
Associate Professor, Department of Radiology,
Ankara Training and Research Hospital,
Ankara, Turkey

Contents

> This article reviews the usefulness of ultrasonography and color Doppler ultrasonography (CDUS) in evaluating children with a suspected renal mass. At ultrasonography, it is possible to locate the site, size, shape, and extent of the mass. Furthermore, the mass can be differentiated as solid or cystic. CDUS helps establish the presence or absence of vascularity in the mass, the relationship with large blood vessels, and presence of thrombus within the renal vein.

> Ultrasonography is the gold standard imaging modality for the assessment of abnormalities of the scrotal contents. Lesions of the paratesticular region in the adult patient are invariably noncancerous, and reassurance is rapidly established. Intratesticular lesions present a diagnostic problem. The presence of a focal intratesticular lesion usually indicates malignant disease, but the importance in establishing the less common benign intratesticular lesion is of paramount importance. Orchidectomy is often performed for these lesions because malignancy cannot be excluded. If identified correctly on ultrasonography, this scenario may be avoided. The article details the common malignant and benign lesions of the scrotal sac and the features of malignant disease and outlines specific features that help the observer identify and establish benign disease to avoid unnecessary surgery.

> Ultrasonography is an important initial imaging modality for the evaluation of the urinary bladder. Distension of the bladder is important for an optimal evaluation of the bladder. Several benign lesions of the bladder, including calculi, diverticula, and ureteroceles, can be detected with ultrasonography. Malignant masses of the bladder can also be diagnosed on ultrasonography based on the internal vascularity, thus differentiating them from blood clots. Some of the other lesions such as colovesical and vesicovaginal fistula are better and more accurately detected on computed tomography or magnetic resonance imaging. Staging of the bladder malignancy also requires additional imaging modalities. Ultrasonography may also have a role in the evaluation of the postoperative bladder.

> Transrectal ultrasonography (TRUS) evaluation has made a significant contribution to the understanding of the diseases affecting the prostate gland, thanks to the advancement in ultrasonography (US) technology during the last 2 decades. Today,

the main indication for TRUS examination of the prostate is the evaluation for prostate cancer and guidance for prostate biopsy. The value of traditional gray-scale TRUS is limited mainly because of variable tumor echogenicity and lower sensitivity and specificity for cancer detection. The visualization of prostate cancer has improved significantly through the use of contrast-enhanced US applications. The final link in the chain is elastography relying on detecting variance in tissue compliance. Although improvements in the accuracy of TRUS provided by the aforementioned encouraging adjuncts are promising, targeted prostate biopsies based on the relevant techniques still cannot preclude the need for systematic biopsies.

Chris J. Harvey and Paul S. Sidhu

Ultrasonography is often the initial imaging modality used in the evaluation of renal diseases. Despite improvements in B mode and Doppler imaging, ultrasonography still has limitations in assessing renal parenchyma because of the heterogeneous echostructure of the cortex and medulla. Ultrasonography also has limitations in the assessment of the renal microcirculation, cortical perfusion and focal masses, and complex cysts. Microbubbles are safe/well-tolerated, pure intravascular agents and can be used in renal failure and obstruction where computed tomography (CT) and magnetic resonance (MR) contrast agents may have deleterious effects. Real-time prolonged imaging can be performed without exposure to ionizing radiation and at a lower cost than CT or MR imaging. This article discusses the European Federation of Societies for Ultrasound in Medicine and Biology guidelines on ultrasound contrast agents and describes how microbubbles can be used to characterize indeterminate renal lesions, complex cysts, and focal inflammatory lesions. Contrast-enhanced ultrasonography is excellent for assessing the renal vasculature and can be used in the diagnosis of renal artery stenosis, renal infarction, renal arterial/venous thrombosis, trauma, as well as the quantification of cortical perfusion. Future applications of microbubbles include the delivery of therapeutic agents and genes.

Ultrasound Clinics

THE CLINICS ARE NOW AVAILABLE ONLINE!

Access your subscription at:
www.theclinics.com

GOAL STATEMENT

The goal of the *Ultrasound Clinics* is to keep practicing radiologists and radiology residents up to date with current clinical practice in ultrasound by providing timely articles reviewing the state of the art in patient care.

ACCREDITATION

The *Ultrasound Clinics* is planned and implemented in accordance with the Essential Areas and Policies of the Accreditation Council for Continuing Medical Education (ACCME) through the joint sponsorship of the University of Virginia School of Medicine and Elsevier. The University of Virginia School of Medicine is accredited by the ACCME to provide continuing medical education for physicians.

The University of Virginia School of Medicine designates this educational activity for a maximum of 15 *AMA PRA Category 1 Credits*™ for each issue, 60 credits per year. Physicians should only claim credit commensurate with the extent of their participation in the activity.

The American Medical Association has determined that physicians not licensed in the US who participate in this CME activity are eligible for a maximum of 15 *AMA PRA Category 1 Credits*™ for each issue, 60 credits per year.

Credit can be earned by reading the text material, taking the CME examination online at http://www.theclinics.com/home/cme, and completing the evaluation. After taking the test, you will be required to review any and all incorrect answers. Following completion of the test and evaluation, your credit will be awarded and you may print your certificate.

FACULTY DISCLOSURE/CONFLICT OF INTEREST

The University of Virginia School of Medicine, as an ACCME accredited provider, endorses and strives to comply with the Accreditation Council for Continuing Medical Education (ACCME) Standards of Commercial Support, Commonwealth of Virginia statutes, University of Virginia policies and procedures, and associated federal and private regulations and guidelines on the need for disclosure and monitoring of proprietary and financial interests that may affect the scientific integrity and balance of content delivered in continuing medical education activities under our auspices.

The University of Virginia School of Medicine requires that all CME activities accredited through this institution be developed independently and be scientifically rigorous, balanced and objective in the presentation/discussion of its content, theories and practices.

All authors/editors participating in an accredited CME activity are expected to disclose to the readers relevant financial relationships with commercial entities occurring within the past 12 months (such as grants or research support, employee, consultant, stock holder, member of speakers bureau, etc.). The University of Virginia School of Medicine will employ appropriate mechanisms to resolve potential conflicts of interest to maintain the standards of fair and balanced education to the reader. Questions about specific strategies can be directed to the Office of Continuing Medical Education, University of Virginia School of Medicine, Charlottesville, Virginia.

The faculty and staff of the University of Virginia Office of Continuing Medical Education have no financial affiliations to disclose.

The authors/editors listed below have identified no professional or financial affiliations for themselves or their spouse/partner:
Matthew J. Bassignani, MD (Test Author); Shweta Bhatt, MD; Vikram S. Dogra, MD (Consulting Editor); Barton Dudlick, (Acquisitions Editor); Chris J. Harvey, MBBS, MRCP, FRCR; Mukund Joshi, MD (Guest Editor); Erkan Kismali, MD; Ashwin Lawande, DNB; Phillip FC Lung, MRCS, FRCR; Ravinder Sidhu, MD; and Ahmet T. Turgut, MD.

The authors/editors listed below have identified the following professional or financial affiliations for themselves or their spouse/partner:
Paul S. Sidhu, MBBS, MRCP, FRCR (Guest Editor) is on the Speakers' Bureau for Bracco (SpA, Milan), Hitachi Japan, and Siemens AG Germany.

Disclosure of Discussion of Non-FDA Approved Uses for Pharmaceutical Products and/or Medical Devices.
The University of Virginia School of Medicine, as an ACCME provider, requires that all faculty presenters identify and disclose any off-label uses for pharmaceutical and medical device products. The University of Virginia School of Medicine recommends that each physician fully review all the available data on new products or procedures prior to clinical use.

TO ENROLL

To enroll in the Ultrasound Clinics Continuing Medical Education program, call customer service at 1-800-654-2452 or visit us online at www.theclinics.com/home/cme. The CME program is available to subscribers for an additional fee of $196.00.

Preface
Genitourinary Ultrasound

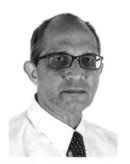
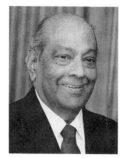

Paul S. Sidhu, MBBS, MRCP, FRCR   Mukund Joshi, MD
Guest Editors

This edition of *Ultrasound Clinics* differs from any preceding issues from the series in one important aspect: we have assembled an array of experts from around the world in order to present the reader with a global and expert view of genitourinary sonography.

Imaging of the genitourinary tract presents many challenges with myriad disease processes presenting with symptoms attributable to the genitourinary system. Sonography remains the first-line imaging procedure and, in many instances, in the child and the neonate, the only imaging modality used. Technical factors related to transducer capabilities, increasing sophistication of computing processing, and the advent of digital imaging have all contributed to a vast improvement in sonographic imaging over the last decade, culminating in the production of exquisite images of diagnostic value. The "discovery" of contrast media that can be used in sonography has revolutionized imaging of the kidneys and is now an accepted technique in many countries where the product is licensed for use (not in the USA yet!). Indeed in the assessment of complex renal cysts and vascular infarction in the transplant kidney may well be regarded as the "gold standard" in the future. Two articles address the use of contrast media in renal disease in the native and transplant kidney.

Imaging the unborn fetus is never easy, and to make a confident interpretation of the many appearances is a great skill to attain. Management is greatly influenced by the findings, and a comprehensive review details the use of sonography in the fetal genitourinary tract. Pediatric diseases of the genitourinary tract are very varied and essentially different from that in the adult, with the renal mass presenting a challenge. A clear understanding is important, with a comprehensive and well-illustrated article addressing this aspect.

In the adult patient, renal infections are often problematic, nearly always in the Western world attributable to a bacterial infection. Not so on a worldwide context where tuberculosis affects the entire genitourinary tract, producing characteristic sonographic features. These two aspects are dealt with in two articles, giving a perspective of infectious diseases affecting the kidneys. Remember that tuberculosis is on the way back in many countries where the disease had all but been eradicated.

Hypertension remains a worldwide problem with severe long-term consequences for the health budget of a country if allowed to cause end-organ damage; it is a "silent" disease. Renal causes are often treatable, and a cost-effective test for this is available with the use of sonography. An article comprehensively covers the diagnosis and pitfalls and reviews the available evidence for the use of sonography to image renal hypertension.

There is often a paucity of information in the literature with regards to male health, which is addressed by articles on the prostate and testis, with a third article on the bladder also presented for good measure. Sonography is the first-line imaging procedure in all three anatomical areas

Ultrasound Clin 5 (2010) ix–x
doi:10.1016/j.cult.2010.10.002

ultrasound.theclinics.com

and often provides a comprehensive view of the abnormalities commonly afflicting these areas. The testis is especially suited to sonography with recourse to other imaging rarely necessary.

Last, minimally invasive techniques are deployed more frequently than ever before to treat diseases of the genitourinary tract, and these procedures are invariably guided by sonography. The skill required to guide intervention by sonography is immense, often underappreciated by clinical colleagues. An article addresses the common procedures in a very practical manner.

It is with great pleasure that we recommend this journal to you, with a wide array of expert reviews from around the world detailing advances, practical aspects, and comprehensively illustrating the many and varied monographic appearances of common, unusual, and rare manifestations of genitourinary disease. We hope you enjoy and benefit from the book.

Paul S. Sidhu, MBBS, MRCP, FRCR
Department of Diagnostic Radiology
King's College Hospital
Denmark Hill
London SE5 9RS, UK

Mukund Joshi, MD
Dr Joshi's Imaging Clinic
809, Harjivandas Estate
Dr Ambedkar Road
Dadar (E) Mumbai 400 014, India

E-mail addresses:
paulsidhu@btinternet.com (P.S. Sidhu)
drmukundjoshi@gmail.com (M. Joshi)

Ultrasonography in Pediatric Renal Masses

Ashwin Lawande, DNB

KEYWORDS

- Ultrasonography • Renal masses
- Color Doppler ultrasonography • Wilms tumor

Ultrasonography is usually the initial modality for imaging for a child with a suspected renal mass. Availability of excellent high-resolution scanners and color Doppler ultrasonography (CDUS) facilities has dramatically changed the diagnostic approach in pediatric patients. Pediatric patients normally have minimal abdominal wall fat and hence ultrasound beam penetration becomes easier. High-frequency curvilinear and linear transducers provide excellent resolution helping to characterize a particular abnormality. The overwhelming attractiveness of pediatric ultrasonography is its real-time imaging ability and its lack of ionizing radiation.

This article reviews the usefulness of ultrasonography and CDUS in evaluating children with a suspected renal mass. At ultrasonography, it is possible to locate the site, size, shape, and extent of the mass. Furthermore, the mass can be differentiated as solid or cystic. CDUS helps in establishing the presence or absence of vascularity in the mass, the relationship with large blood vessels, and the presence of thrombus within the renal vein.

NORMAL SONOGRAPHIC ANATOMY OF THE KIDNEY

Neonatal and infant kidneys have a different appearance from the kidneys of older children (**Fig. 1**). In infants, the echogenicity of renal cortex is increased and usually equal to or slightly greater than that of the adjacent liver or spleen. In older children, the cortex is hypoechoic relative to these structures. This is thought due to the increased

relative number and cellularity of the glomeruli, leading to more acoustic interfaces in infants.[1] The medullary pyramids are hypoechoic and prominent in neonates and infants because they have smaller cortical volume as compared with older children. The ratio of cortex to medulla is 1.64:1 in neonates compared with 2.59:1 in adults.[1,2] The echogenicity of the central sinus is slighter in neonates and infants compared with adolescents due to the increase in renal sinus fat as the age advances.[1,2]

NORMAL VARIANTS

It is of particular importance in children to recognize a normal variant to avoid misinterpretation as a renal mass.

Fetal Lobulation and Column of Bertin

The normal kidney is formed from fusion of multiple lobes. These lobulations form an undulating margin along the cortical border, which sometimes persist in postnatal life (**Fig. 2**).[3] The adjacent cortices of contiguous renal lobes fuse to form a thick layer of cortex, termed a column of Bertin. A column of Bertin has echogenicity equal to or slightly higher than the cortex, extending from the interpyramidal region and projecting into the renal sinus.[4] Ultrasonography demonstrates continuity with the renal cortex, and on CDUS and power Doppler, a vascular pattern identical to the normal renal parenchyma is demonstrated (**Fig. 3**).[5]

Dr Joshi's Imaging Clinic, 809 Harjivandas Estate, Dr Ambedkar Road, Dadar TT, Mumbai 400014, Maharashtra, India
E-mail address: ashlawande@yahoo.co.in

Ultrasound Clin 5 (2010) 433–441
doi:10.1016/j.cult.2010.07.003
1556-858X/10/$ — see front matter © 2010 Published by Elsevier Inc.

ultrasound.theclinics.com

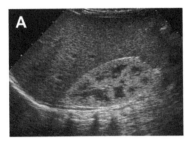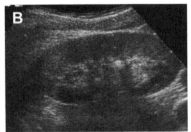

Fig. 1. (*A*) Normal pediatric kidney. The cortex appears hyperechogenic compared with adjacent liver or spleen. The renal pyramids appear more prominent in comparison with normal adult kidney. (*B*) Normal adult kidney for comparison.

Dromedary Hump

A dromedary hump is a bulge in the lateral margin of the midpole of the left kidney due to the extrinsic impression by the spleen on the upper half of the kidney. A dromedary hump has the appearance of normal renal parenchyma and CDUS demonstrates normal vascular architecture (**Fig. 4**).

Junctional Parenchymal Defect

A junctional parenchymal defect appears as a triangular echogenic focus near the junction of the upper and middle thirds of the kidney. A junctional parenchymal defect and inter-renicular septum represent the plane of fusion of renal lobes. The septum is seen as a thin echogenic line connecting the junctional parenchymal defect with the renal sinus (**Fig. 5**).[6,7]

RENAL MASSES

Renal masses are the most common abdominal masses in neonates, infants, and older children. In neonates and infants, most renal masses are usually benign, the most common being hydronephrosis.[8] In older children, malignant masses are more common.

Benign Renal Masses

Congenital hydronephrosis

Congenital hydronephrosis is the most common benign renal mass in neonates and infants. The most common cause is a pelviureteric junction (PUJ) obstruction.[9] The degree of dilatation is dependent on the severity and duration of obstruction. The cause is controversial but is believed due to abnormal development of the ureteral smooth muscle at the PUJ. Extrinsic factors, such as bands, adhesions, or aberrant vessels, have also been implicated. The characteristic ultrasonographic findings include multiple cystic structures of uniform size (dilated calyces) communicating with each other and with a larger cystic structure that represents the renal pelvis (**Fig. 6**). There is renal parenchyma of varying thickness seen around these cystic areas with no visualization of the upper ureter. Chronic severe obstruction can lead to thinning and dysplastic changes in the renal parenchyma. The parenchyma becomes

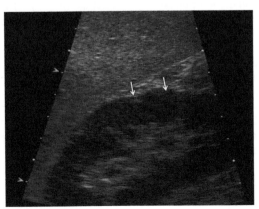

Fig. 2. Fetal lobulations (*arrows*). Persistent lobulated margins of the renal cortex due to fusion of embryonic renunculi.

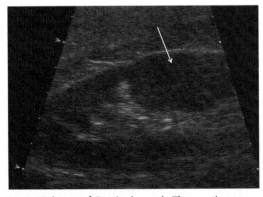

Fig. 3. Column of Bertin (*arrow*). The contiguous renunculi fuse to form a thick band of cortical echogenicity without any cortical bulge, seen to extend from renal sinus up to medulla.

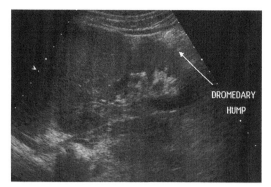

Fig. 4. Dromedary hump (*arrow*) seen most often at midregion with echogenicity identical to that of the renal cortex and contains normal renal pyramids within.

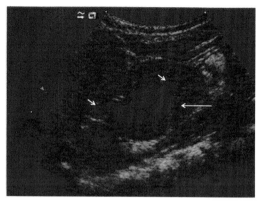

Fig. 6. PUJ obstruction. There is dilatation of pelvicalyceal system with parenchymal thinning. The pelvis (*long arrow*) appears more dilated than calyces (*short arrows*), with no visualization of a dilated proximal ureter.

echogenic and sometimes shows degenerative cysts. Rupture of renal collecting system leads to urinary leak resulting in subcapsular urinomas or ascites. On serial follow-up imaging, a measurement of the anteroposterior dimension of the renal pelvis (best on axial kidney view) is recorded along with the parenchymal thickness. Normally a child undergoes surgical intervention (pyeloplasty) based on the function of the kidney on scintigraphy; a functioning kidney is salvaged. Postpyeloplasty, a mild residual dilatation persists but the function of the kidney shows significant improvement. CDUS can sometimes demonstrate aberrant vessels crossing the PUJ.

Renal cystic disease

Autosomal recessive polycystic kidney disease Autosomal recessive polycystic kidney disease is a congenital abnormality affecting both kidneys, inherited as a recessive characteristic. The kidneys are enlarged, show multiple minute (1–2 mm) cysts in the cortex and medulla,

and are associated with hepatic fibrosis.[10–12] On ultrasonography in neonates with autosomal recessive polycystic kidney disease, both kidneys are enlarged and diffusely echogenic with poor differentiation of the renal sinus, medulla, and cortex (**Fig. 7**).[13,14] The hyperechogenicity of the kidney is due to multiple fluid and cyst wall interfaces. An echo-poor rim is seen in 50% of cases along the periphery, which could be due to a compressed normal renal cortex or fluid-filled, thin-walled cystic spaces in subcapsular region (see **Fig. 7**).[13,15,16] In older children, the disease may be a slightly milder form with normal to enlarged kidneys, showing hypoechoic cortex and prominent echogenic pyramids.[15,16] The fibrosis in the liver varies with age; in older patients, there is an increase in periportal fibrosis,

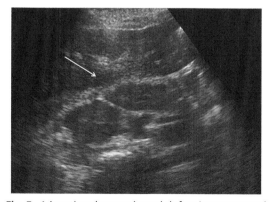

Fig. 5. A junctional parenchymal defect is represented by a thin echogenic septum (*arrow*) seen at upper and middle third of the kidney.

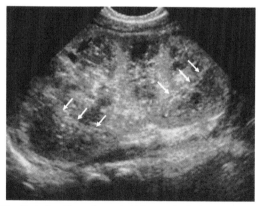

Fig. 7. Infantile polycystic kidney. The kidney appears echogenic and enlarged in size with thin hypoehoic peripheral rim representing normal compressed renal parenchyma (*white arrows*). The black arrow points to a cystic space.

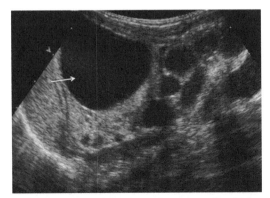

Fig. 8. MCDK. Unilateral involvement of a kidney showing bright cortex, loss of corticomedullary differentiation, and multiple cysts. The dominant cyst (*arrow*) most often is eccentrically located along the lateral margin of the kidney. Such kidney is nonfunctional.

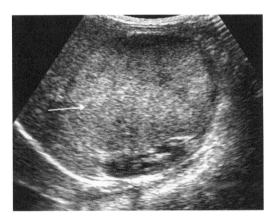

Fig. 10. Mesoblastic nephroma. A large well defined homogenous mass (*arrow*) occupying the renal region with no evidence of corticomedullary differentiation.

diffusely increased parenchymal echogenicity, and findings of portal hypertension.

Multicystic dysplastic kidney disease Multicystic dysplastic kidney (MCDK) disease is normally unilateral and involves a severe form of renal dysplasia. An early in utero obstruction within the first 10 weeks causes atresia of the renal pelvis and proximal ureter, leading to MCDK.[17] An insult after 10 weeks results in a hydronephrotic form. On ultrasonography, there are multiple noncommunicating cysts of varying sizes with an intervening echogenic dysplastic parenchyma (**Fig. 8**). There is no differentiation between the cortex, medulla, and renal sinus fat. Most of these kidneys undergo regression and atrophy in the first 2 years of life; hence, they are managed conservatively unless complications, such as infection or

hypertension, arise.[18] Approximately 20% to 50% of infants with MCDK have a contralateral vesicoureteral reflux, duplication anomalies, and PUJ obstruction.[15,19,20] If the MCDK is managed conservatively, serial imaging studies are mandatory due to slightly increased incidence of Wilms tumor.[21] It is often difficult to differentiate MCDK from a cystic Wilms tumor or a cystic renal cell carcinoma (RCC).

Multilocular cystic nephroma Multilocular cystic nephroma is an uncommon, benign, sporadic neoplasm with a biphasic age and gender distribution, seen in boys younger than 2 years of age and in women older than 30 years of age.[22,23] On ultrasonography, there is a well-defined multicystic, septated mass seen with septa of varying thickness. Any solid component along the septa is suspicious for malignancy. The loculations may

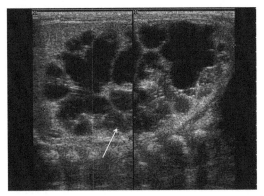

Fig. 9. Multilocular cystic nephroma. Multiple cysts of varying size with septations and internal echoes representing either hemorrhage or mucoid material (*arrow*).

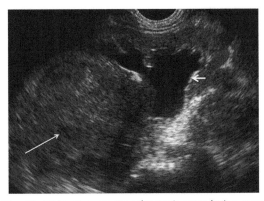

Fig. 11. Wilms tumor. An echogenic mass lesion seen arising from upper pole of the kidney (*long arrow*) causing pelvicalyceal obstruction (*short arrow*).

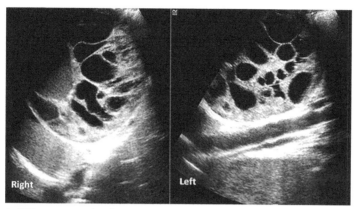

Fig. 12. Bilateral cystic Wilms tumors closely resembling a multicystic nephroma. There are multiple noncommunicating cysts with thickened septations.

not be evident if there is hemorrhage or mucoid material within the cystic components (**Fig. 9**).[22,23]

Mesoblastic nephroma

Mesoblastic nephroma, also termed *mesenchymal hamartoma*, is the most common solid renal mass in infants, with a slight male predominance.[24] A mesoblastic nephroma presents as a painless abdominal mass, less frequently with hematuria. On histology, the tumor is a solid unencapsulated mass believed to consist of early nephrogenic mesenchyme, somewhat similar to a uterine leiomyoma.[25,26] On ultrasonography, there is usually a large echogenic mass with a homogenous echo pattern. On occasion, the mass demonstrates a heterogeneous echo texture with areas of necrosis and hemorrhage. A mesoblastic nephroma has a tendency for perinephric invasion but usually does not involve the renal vessels or the renal pelvis.[26] Because this is a benign tumor, a nephrectomy alone suffices but a wider surgical margin is necessary due to the often-present infiltrative findings. Rarely, the lesion may recur locally or, if incompletely resected, may metastasize to the lungs, brain or bones (**Fig. 10**).[27]

Angiomyolipomas

Angiomyolipomas are common benign lesions in adults but rarely seen in children. They appear as well-defined echogenic mass due to intracellular fat. Approximately 80% to 85% of angiomyolipomas are associated with tuberous sclerosis.

Malignant Renal Masses

Wilms tumor

Wilms tumor is the most common primary renal neoplasm in children, accounting for 87% of pediatric renal masses, and occurs in approximately 1:10,000 children.[28,29] The diagnosis is made most often in children younger than 5 years of age. The child commonly presents with a palpable abdominal mass. Hypertension is seen in 90% of patients either due to renin production by the tumor or to compression of hilar vessels. Other

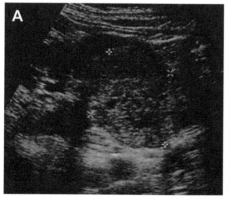
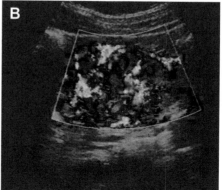

Fig. 13. Wilms tumor. (*A*) An echogenic mass at the lower aspect of the left kidney (between cursors). (*B*) There is marked increase in the CDUS signal from the mass lesion.

symptoms include abdominal pain, hematuria, and fever. Clinical syndromes or anomalies associated with Wilms tumor include sporadic aniridia, cryptorchidism, hemihypertrophy, Beckwith-Wiedmann syndrome, and Drash syndrome.[30–32] Wilms tumor can also arise in a horseshoe kidney, MCDK, and extrarenal sites, such as the inguinal canal, sacrococcygeal region, genital structures, retroperitoneum, and chest wall.[33–35]

On histology, Wilms tumor is sharply delineated by a pseudocapsule composed of compressed renal tissue, with 90% of these tumors demonstrating a favorable histology (ie, primitive blastomal, stromal, and epithelial elements). The remaining 10% have anaplastic elements conferring an unfavorable histology, with contiguous spread to adjacent tissues and distant metastasis to lung, liver, bone, or brain.[30,32]

On ultrasonography, the visualized renal mass and related structures may have the following features:

A predominantly echogenic mass (**Fig. 11**)
Homogeneity or heterogeneity depending on the areas of hemorrhage, necrosis, fat, or calcification, with cystic change also seen (**Fig. 12**)
A sharp parenchymal interface
Pseudocapsule
Renal vein or inferior vena cava (IVC) thrombosis
Enlarged lymph nodes
CDUS showing tumor neovascularity and sometimes arteriovenous shunting (**Fig. 13**).

Spread to hilar or retroperitoneal lymph nodes occurs in 20% of cases. The liver is most common abdominal organ involved by metastasis (10% patients). Extracapsular involvement and lymph node and distant metastases are better evaluated by CT or MR imaging.[36,37] **Box 1** details the staging classification of Wilms tumor.

Prognosis depends on the histologic cell type. Well-differentiated tumors have better prognosis than the anaplastic type. Nephrectomy with adjuvant chemotherapy is dnormally performed. Presurgical chemotherapy is used for tumor shrinkage and local radiation therapy of tumor bed is performed in the postoperative period when there is gross spillage of tumor identified at the time of surgery.

Nephroblastomatosis

Nephroblastomatosis is an abnormality characterized by persistence of fetal renal blastema beyond 36 weeks of gestation. Nephroblastomatosis may be classified as perilobar or intralobar on the basis

---

Box 1
Staging of Wilms tumor

Stage and features

I. Confined to the kidney with an intact capsule
II. Local spread beyond the kidney, which can be resected
III. Residual disease confined to abdomen

   Nonhematogenous includes

   a. Positive abdominal nodes
   b. Diffuse peritoneal contamination
   c. Positive margins
   d. Residual nonresected tumor

IV. Hematogenous spread to distant organs, such as lungs, liver, or nodes
V. Bilateral disease; each side should be staged separately because prognosis is dependent on the individual stage

Data from White KS, Grossman H. Wilms' and associated renal tumors of childhood. Pediatr Radiol 1991;21:81–8.

---

of location. Nephroblastomatosis is thought to be a precursor to malignant transformation to Wilms tumor.[38] Thirty percent to 40% of Wilms tumors arise from these nephrogenic rests, with foci of nephroblastomatosis seen in almost 99% of bilateral Wilms tumors. These foci are also present in Beckwith-Wiedmann syndrome, hemihypertrophy and sporadic aniridia, Perlman syndrome, and trisomy 18, all conditions with a predilection to developing a Wilms tumor. On ultrasonography,

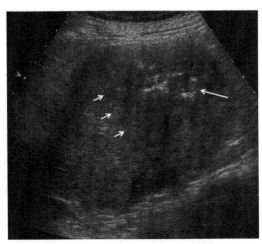

Fig. 14. RCC. A heterogeneous irregular mass (*small arrows*) arising in the left kidney, with focal areas of high reflectivity (*long arrow*) in keeping with calcification.

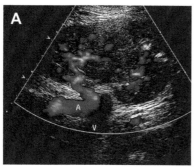
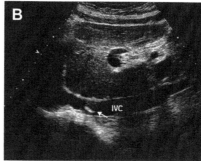

Fig. 15. RCC. (*A*) A power Doppler image of a left kidney involved with an RCC. The renal artery is patent (A) whereas there is no flow in the renal vein (V), indicating thrombosis of the vein. (*B*) B-mode image showing thrombosis (*arrow*) in the IVC.

the kidney is enlarged but maintains its reniform shape. Diffuse disease presents as a peripheral rind of hypoechoic tissue. Corticomedullary differentiation is absent. Focal disease presents as a hypoechoic mass and when present in a subcapsular location is highly suggestive of nephroblastomatosis.[38,39]

Renal cell carcinoma

RCC is rare in children, accounting for less than 7% of all primary renal tumors manifesting in the first two decades of life. The peak incidence is in adults, in the sixth decade; less than 2% of cases occur in pediatric patients.[40] In von Hippel-Lindau disease, the tumors are multiple and affect younger adults and children. Clinically, patients present with gross painless hematuria, flank pain, and a palpable mass. On histology, an RCC is an adenocarcinoma with renal tubular differentiation, normally smaller than a Wilms tumor, and forms an infiltrating solid mass with variable necrosis, hemorrhage, calcification, and cystic degeneration. There is often a pseudocapsule present. Local spread occurs to the adjacent retroperitoneum and lymph nodes. Distant metastases to lungs, bones, liver, and brain are seen in 20% of patients.[24] On ultrasonography, the tumors are solid with a homogenous or a heterogenous appearance. Calcification is seen in one-third of these tumors (**Fig. 14**).[41,42] Vascular invasion into the renal vein and IVC often occurs in advanced disease (**Fig. 15**). CDUS may show the vascularity of the tumor and ascertain the presence of vascular involvement. Sometimes, small tumors are difficult to detect and are better identified with CT or MR imaging. There is a higher frequency of calcification in RCC (25%) than in Wilms tumors (9%).[38] The standard treatment is radical nephrectomy with regional lymphadenectomy, with an overall survival rate of approximately 64%. The tumor is resistant to chemotherapy.

Renal lymphoma

Renal involvement is usually a late manifestation of lymphoma present elsewhere. Renal involvement is seen in non-Hodgkin lymphoma, especially Burkitt lymphoma. Primary renal lymphoma is unlikely because there is no lymphoid tissue in the kidney. On ultrasonography, there is focal or diffuse involvement. There may be solid hypoechoic renal masses seen or, more often, there is diffuse enlargement of the kidney with a grossly hypoechoic thickened parenchyma compressing the sinus echoes. In secondary lymphomatous involvement of kidney, there is thickening of Gerota's fascia with regional lymphadenopathy (**Fig. 16**).[43,44]

Renal leukemia

Renal involvement in leukemia, as in lymphoma, is a late manifestation of the disease. There is generally diffuse bilateral renal involvement. On ultrasonography, both kidneys are enlarged with

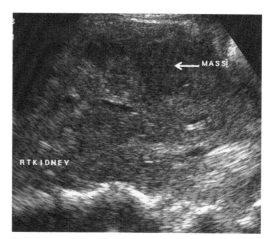

Fig. 16. Renal lymphoma. A mass (*arrow*) in a subcapsular position, of secondary renal involvement with lymphoma.

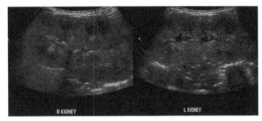

Fig. 17. Renal leukemia. Bilateral enlarged kidneys with loss of corticomedullary differentiation.

increased cortical echogenicity. The corticomedullary differentiation is lost (**Fig. 17**).

Clear cell sarcoma

Clear cell sarcoma is a rare primary renal tumor with a male predominance, accounting for 4% to 5% of pediatric renal tumors, and has a peak incidence at 1 to 4 years of age. Clear cell sarcoma has been termed the bone-metastasizing renal tumor of childhood.[24] Although histopathologic appearances are characteristic, the imaging studies cannot differentiate a clear cell sarcoma from a Wilms tumor. A clear cell sarcoma is usually a solid renal mass, which may show varying degree of echogenicity depending on the amount of necrosis or hemorrhage. There is higher incidence of recurrence and mortality due to aggressive behavior as compared with Wilms tumor, with spread to the bones, lymph nodes, brain, liver, and lungs. Nephrectomy and chemotherapy are the modes of treatment, with long-term survival rates of 60% to 70%.

Rhabdoid tumor

Rhabdoid tumors are a rare, highly aggressive, malignant renal tumors in the pediatric age group. The majority (80%) of these tumors occur at less than 2 years of age with a male predominance.[24] A rhabdoid tumor has a histologic appearance resembling a tumor of skeletal muscle origin; however, a myogenic origin has not been proved. There is an association of rhabdoid tumor with primary intracranial masses or brain metastases. There may be hypercalcemia secondary to elevated parathyroid hormone levels.[45] On ultrasonography, there is usually a large centrally located mass with a heterogenous appearance that is difficult to differentiate from a Wilms tumor; however, certain features, such as subcapsular fluid collections, tumor nodules separated by areas of necrosis, and hemorrhage, are often seen. Calcifications can also be seen in these nodules, with local and vascular invasion common.[24,45,46] Because this tumor is highly aggressive and metastasizes early, it has the worst prognosis of all pediatric renal tumors. Overall survival rate is poor, as low as 20% at 18 months' post diagnosis.[46] The most common metastasizing site is lung followed by the liver, abdomen, brain, lymph nodes, and bone.

SUMMARY

Ultrasonography is a safe, portable, and inexpensive imaging modality for the evaluation of pediatric masses. Ultrasonography helps diagnose and characterize renal mass lesion and can serve as guide for biopsies in real time. Wilms tumor is the most common pediatric solid renal neoplasm, with several other renal masses recognized as separate pathologic entities, which can be diagnosed with ultrasonography. Knowledge of the many distinct clinical and ultrasonographic imaging features helps suggest a particular diagnosis.

REFERENCES

1. Han BK, Babcock DS. Sonographic measurements and appearance of normal kidneys in children. AJR Am J Roentgenol 1985;145:611–6.
2. Vade A, Lau P, Smick J, et al. Sonographic renal parameters as related to age. Pediatr Radiol 1987; 17:212–5.
3. Patriquin H, Lefaivre JF, Lafortune M, et al. Fetal lobation: an anatomo-ultrasonographic correlation. J Ultrasound Med 1990;9:191–7.
4. Lafortune M, Constantin A, Breton G, et al. Sonography of the hypertrophied column of Bertin. AJR Am J Roentgenol 1986;146:53–6.
5. Ascenti G, Zimbaro G, Mazziotti S, et al. Contrast-enhanced power Doppler US in the diagnosis of renal pseudotumors. Eur Radiol 2001;11:2496–9.
6. Tsushima Y, Sato N, Ishizaka H, et al. US findings of junctional parenchymal defect of the kidney. Nippon Igaku Hoshasen Gakkai Zasshi 1992;52:436–42.
7. Hoffer FA, Hanobergh AM, Teele RL. The interrenicular junction: a mimic of renal scarring on normal pediatric sonograms. AJR Am J Roentgenol 1985; 145:1075–8.
8. Woodard JR. Hydronephrosis in the neonate. Urology 1993;42:620–1.
9. Brown T, Mandell J, Lebowitz RL. Neonatal hydronephrosis in the era of sonography. AJR Am J Roentgenol 1987;148:959–63.
10. Hartman DS. Renal cystic disease in multisystem conditions. Urol Radiol 1992;14:13–7.
11. Madewell JE, Hartman DS, Litchtenstein JR. Radiologic- pathologic correlation in cystic diseases of the kidney. Radiol Clin North Am 1979;17:261–79.
12. Premkumar A, Berdon WE, Levy J, et al. The emergence of hepatic fibrosis and portal hypertension in infants and children with autosomal recessive

polycystic kidney disease: initial and follow up sonographic and radiographic findings. Pediatr Radiol 1988;18:123–9.

13. Hayden CK Jr, Swischuk LE. Renal cystic disease. Semin Ultrasound CT MR 1991;12:361–73.

14. Jain M, Lequesne GW, Bourne AJ, et al. High resolution ultrasonography in the differential diagnosis of cystic diseases of the kidney in infancy and childhood: preliminary experience. J Ultrasound Med 1997;16:235–40.

15. Blickman JG, Bramson RT, Herrin JT. Autosomal recessive polycystic kidney disease: long term sonographic findings in patients surviving the neonatal period. AJR Am J Roentgenol 1995;164:1247–50.

16. Harman TE, Siegel MJ. Pyramidal hyperechogenicity in autosomal recessive polycystic kidney disease resembling medullary nephrocalcinosis. Pediatr Radiol 1991;21:270–1.

17. Beck AD. The effect of intrauterine urinary obstruction upon the development of the fetal kidney. J Urol 1971;105:784–9.

18. Rottenberg GT, Gordon I, De Bruyn R. The natural history of MCDK in children. Br J Radiol 1997;70: 347–50.

19. Flack CE, Bellinger MF. The multicystic dysplastic kidney and contralateral vesicoureteral reflux: protection of the solitary kidney. J Urol 1993;150:1873–4.

20. Karmazyn B, Zerin JM. Lower urinary tract abnormalities in children with multicystic dysplastic kidney. Radiology 1997;203:223–6.

21. Hartman GE, Smolik LM, Shochat SJ. The dilemma of the multicystic dysplastic kidney. Am J Dis child 1986;140:925–8.

22. Agrons GA, Wagner BJ, Davidson AJ, et al. Multilocular cystic renal tumor in children: radiologic-pathologic correlation. Radiographics 1995;16: 653–69.

23. Gervais DA, Whitman GJ, Chew FS. Multilocular cyst of the kidney. AJR Am J Roentgenol 1993;161:600.

24. Gellen E, Smergel EM, Lowry PA. Renal neoplasms of childhood. Radiol Clin North Am 1997;35:1391–413.

25. Simonton SC, Dehner LP. The kidney and lower urinary tract. In: Stocker JT, Dehner LP, editors. Pediatric pathology, vol. 2. 3rd edition. Philadelphia: JB Lippincott; 1992. p. 719–21, 11

26. Wooten SL, Rowen SJ, Griscom NT. Congenital mesoblastic nephroma. Radiographics 1991;11: 719–21.

27. Lowe LH, Isuani BH, Heller RM, et al. Pediatric renal masses: Wilm's tumor and beyond. Radiographics 2000;20:1585–603.

28. Julian JC, Mergnerian PA, Shortliffe LMD. Pediatric genitourinary tumors. Curr Opin Oncol 1995;7: 265–74.

29. Ritchey ML, Azizphan RG, Bekwith JB, et al. Neonatal Wilms tumor. J Pediatr Surg 1995;30: 856–9.

30. Green DM, Goppes MJ, Brestow NE, et al. Wilm's tumor. In: Pizzo PA, Poplack DG, editors. Principles and practice of pediatric oncology. 3rd edition. New York: Lippincott – Raven; 1997. p. 733–59.

31. Paterson A, Sweeney LE. Teratoid Wilms' tumor occurring synchronously with classical Wilm's tumor in Beckwith Wiedemann syndrome. Pediatr Radiol 2000;30:656–7.

32. White KS, Grossman H. Wilms' and associated renal tumors of childhood. Pediatr Radiol 1991;21:81–8.

33. Broecrer BH, Caldamone AA, McWilliams NB, et al. Primary extrarenal Wilm's tumor in children. J Pediatr Surg 1989;24:1283–8.

34. Navoy JF, Royal SA, Vaid YN, et al. Wilm's tumor: unusual manifestations. Pediatr Radiol 1995;25: S76–86.

35. Song JH, Hansen K, Wallach MT. Extrarenal Wilm's tumor. J Ultrasound Med 1997;16:149–51.

36. Cremin BJ. Wilm's tumor: ultrasound and changing concepts. Clin Radiol 1987;38:465–74.

37. Reiman TH, Siegel MJ, Shackelford GD. Wilm's tumor in children: abdominal CT and US evaluation. Radiology 1986;160:501–5.

38. Lonergan GJ, Mastinez – Leon MI, Agrons GA, et al. Nephrogenic rest, nephroblastomatosis and associated lesions of the kidney. Radiographics 1998;18: 947–68.

39. Gallant JM, Barnemolt CE, Taylor GA, et al. Radiologic—pathologic conference of children's hospital Boston: bilateral asymptomatic renal enlargement. Pediatr Radiol 1997;27:614–7.

40. Lack EE, Cassady JR, Sallan SE. Renal cell carcinoma in childhood and adolescence: a clinical and pathological study of 17 cases. J Urol 1985;133:822–8.

41. Kabala JE, Shield J, Duncan A. Renal cell carcinoma in childhood. Pediatr Radiol 1992;22:203–5.

42. Sostre G, Johnson JF III, Cho M. Ossifying renal cell carcinoma. Pediatr Radiol 1998;28:458–60.

43. Mcguire PM, Merrif CRB, Ducos RS. Ultrasonography of primary renal lymphoma in a child. J Ultrasound Med 1996;15:479–81.

44. Weinberger E, Rosenbaum DM, Pendergrass TW. Renal involvement in children with lymphoma: comparison of CT with sonography. AJR Am J Roentgenol 1990;155:347–9.

45. Agrons GA, Kingsman KD, Wagner BJ, et al. Rhabdoid tumors of the kidney in children: a comparative study. AJR Am J Roentgenol 1997;168:447–51.

46. Chung CJ, Lorenzo R, Rayder S, et al. Rhabdoid tumors of the kidney in children: CT findings. AJR Am J Roentgenol 1995;164:697–700.

Ultrasonography for Scrotal Masses, Benign and Malignant

Phillip FC. Lung, MRCS, FRCR, Paul S. Sidhu, MBBS, MRCP, FRCR*

KEYWORDS

- Scrotal mass • Testicular tumor • Testicular torsion
- Scrotal inflammation

A testicular mass on ultrasonography, whether an incidental finding or when the adult patient presents with a "lump," has profound implications for the patient. Most intratesticular masses are malignant and require an orchidectomy, further imaging, and probably chemotherapy. Some intratesticular abnormalities are benign, many with particular ultrasonographic features that point to the benign nature. Extratesticular lesions, nearly always benign in the adult patient, cause considerable patient anxiety; ultrasound examination confirms the benign nature and offers instant patient reassurance. This article details the many scrotal masses encountered in daily practice, allowing the examiner to have a comprehensive overview of the subject to improve confidence in arriving at the correct diagnosis.

ANATOMY

During fetal development, the testes pass into the scrotal sac with a covering of dense fibrous connective tissue, the tunica albuginea. A fold of the processus vaginalis envelops the testes during its descent through the inguinal canal, becoming the visceral layer of the tunica vaginalis, while the parietal layer lines the scrotal sac. The testes and associated structures are separated from each other by a midline septum. The scrotal sac itself is arranged in layers, which are the internal spermatic fascia (deepest layer), cremasteric fascia, external spermatic fascia, dartos muscle, superficial fascia, and the skin (superficial layer).

The posterior tunica albuninea extends into the testis to form the mediastinum, which divides the testis into lobules via fibrous septa. Each lobule contains seminiferous tubules, Sertoli cells, and spermatocytes that are responsible for sperm production. Testosterone is produced by the Leydig cells that are embedded into the interstitium of the tubules. The seminiferous tubules open into the rete testis within the mediastinum, which then drains into the epididymis.

The crescent-shaped epididymis lies adjacent to the posterior aspect of the testis and consists of a head (located superiorly), body, and tail. Approximately 10 efferent ducts make up the epididymal head, and these eventually coalesce into a single duct in the body and tail, which finally becomes the vas deferens.

The scrotal sac and its contents are supplied by (1) the testicular artery, which originates from the aorta and supplies the testis; (2) the cremasteric artery, which arises from the inferior epigastric artery and supplies the scrotum and spermatic cord layers; and (3) the artery to the vas deferens. The veins draining the testis and epididymis converge to form the pampiniform plexus at the superior pole of the testis. This continues as the testicular vein, which drains into the inferior vena cava on the right and the left renal vein on the left.

ULTRASOUND ANATOMY

The testicular echo texture is homogeneous and of intermediate reflectivity. A hyperechoic linear structure runs in the longitudinal plane of each testis, representing the mediastinum testis; this drains the seminiferous tubules into the rete testis. The rete testis is located at the testicular hilum and

Department of Radiology, King's College Hospital, Denmark Hill, London SE5 9RS, UK
* Corresponding author.
E-mail address: paulsidhu@nhs.net

Ultrasound Clin 5 (2010) 443–456
doi:10.1016/j.cult.2010.05.002

appears hypoechoic with projections into the parenchyma. Testicular volume (of both testes) exceeding 30 mL is in keeping with normal testicular function. Vascular perfusion can be investigated using color Doppler ultrasonography or power Doppler ultrasonography. Normal intratesticular color Doppler flow can be reliably detected with a testicular volume greater than 2 mL.[1]

SCROTAL WALL ABNORMALITIES

Scrotal wall abnormalities can be broadly categorized into those with inflammatory or noninflammatory causes. The noninflammatory causes for scrotal wall edema may be general, such as cardiac, hepatic, or renal failure, or more local, including postoperative causes, venous obstruction, and lymphoedema (**Fig. 1**).

Scrotal Wall Cellulitis

The cause for inflammation is mostly infection, with scrotal wall cellulitis being more common in susceptible patients, such as those who are diabetic or immunocompromised. The ultrasonographic appearances of cellulitis are thickening of the subcutaneous layer and increased heterogeneity, with increased color Doppler flow. It is important to identify developing abscess formation, which are seen as well-defined, irregular hypoechoic lesions within the scrotal wall, as the abscess may require drainage.

Fournier Gangrene

Fournier gangrene (**Fig. 2**) is a polymicrobial necrotizing fasciitis of the perineal and genital regions, characterized by a rapid rate of progression and a high mortality rate ranging from 15% to 50%.[2] Although computed tomography remains

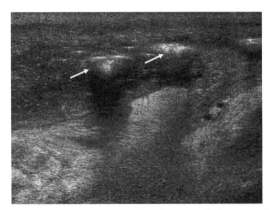

Fig. 2. In this patient with infection of the scrotal skin, areas of high reflectivity (*arrows*) represent air in Fournier gangrene.

the imaging modality of choice, ultrasonography can provide important evidence in the undiagnosed patient. Scrotal wall thickening is present, with hyperechoic foci causing reverberation artifact, which indicates subcutaneous gas and is characteristic of Fournier gangrene.[3] An important diagnostic differential is strangulated bowel within an inguinal hernia and can be distinguished by gas in the bowel wall and not in the scrotal wall.

ABNORMALITIES OF THE TUNICA VAGINALIS
Hydrocele

A hydrocele is the most common cause of painless scrotal swelling and the ultrasonographic appearances are usually of an anechoic fluid collection seen around the testis, although low-level echoes may occasionally be demonstrated.[4] Hydroceles are serous fluid collections and can be congenital or acquired. The congenital form involves incomplete closure of the processus vaginalis, allowing fluid to be transmitted from the peritoneal cavity; this places patients at increased risk of developing an inguinal hernia. Acquired hydroceles may be idiopathic or secondary to various factors, such as infection or tumor. A "snow-storm" hydrocele (**Fig. 3**) has been attributed to cholesterol crystals or a high protein content that produces florid "swirling" echoes.[5] Up to 86% of asymptomatic men display a small amount of fluid between the visceral and parietal layers of the tunica vaginalis.[6]

Hematocele and Pyocele

It is important to distinguish a hydrocele from other causes of fluid within tunica vaginalis: hematoceles, usually secondary to trauma or surgery, and pyoceles, most often occurring because of untreated epididymo-orchitis. Hematoceles often present with scrotal discomfort and a hard scrotal

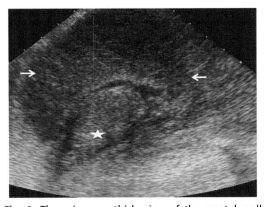

Fig. 1. There is gross thickening of the scrotal wall (*arrows*) in a patient with advanced scrotal edema secondary to cardiac failure. The underlying testis is normal (*star*).

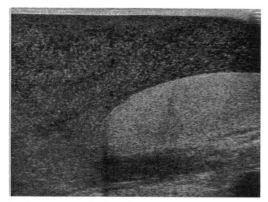

Fig. 3. A chronic hydrocele is present with echogenic debris within representing cholesterol crystals.

mass with a complex heterogeneous appearance and may demonstrate mass effect with distortion of the testis. Pyoceles present with acute scrotal pain and symptoms of sepsis. A pyocele (**Fig. 4**) also appears heterogeneous on the ultrasonogram, and gas may be identified, causing hyperechoic reflections and shadowing.

PARATESTICULAR LESIONS
Inguinal Hernia

An inguinal hernia is a common paratesticular mass and is usually diagnosed by clinical history and examination but are often referred for imaging. Inguinal hernias are classified as being indirect, having to pass through the deep inguinal ring, or direct, traversing through the anterior wall musculature. The relationship of these hernias with the inferior epigastric artery can be exploited during ultrasonography; the hernia is indirect if the neck of the hernia is lateral to this landmark and direct

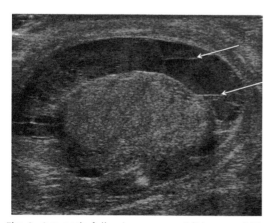

Fig. 4. A pyocele following severe epididymo-orchitis. Septations (*arrows*) are present in the echogenic infected fluid surrounding the testis.

if the inferior epigastric artery lies medially. The hernial sac most commonly contains bowel, which can be positively diagnosed if peristalsis can be demonstrated, or omentum, which may be mistaken for a lipoma. Rarer contents include a Meckel's diverticulum and part of the urinary bladder. An important consideration is bowel strangulation, which is a surgical emergency, and may be positively identified by a nonperistalsing dilated loop of bowel; this has been reported to have a sensitivity of 90% and specificity of 93%.[7] Bowel contains gas and fluid, producing acoustic shadowing and enhancement, respectively, which can be mistaken for an abscess, although clinical history should favor one or the other.

Splenogonadal Fusion

Splenunculi represent congenital splenic tissue that is separate from the body of the spleen and is found in 10% to 30% of patients at autopsy.[8] Splenogonadal fusion is a rare abnormality described as the fusion of an accessory spleen to the gonads, ovary or testis. Splenogonadal fusion, in the male patient, presents as a painless scrotal mass and is associated with cryptorchidism and an inguinal hernia. Two types are recognized: the more common continuous type, whereby a cord connects the splenunculus to the spleen, and the discontinuous type, without a cord. B-mode appearances are of a homogeneous mass, which is more hypoechoic compared with the testicular parenchyma, and is contiguous with the spleen. This malformation may be differentiated from testicular malignancy with color Doppler ultrasonography, in which a central branching vascular pattern may be seen extending to the periphery, as opposed to the disorganized pattern observed in cancer.[9] The diagnosis is confirmed with a technetium Tc 99m sulfur colloid study, which demonstrates similar uptake within the spleen and testicular splenunculus, thus avoiding unnecessary orchidectomy.[10]

SPERMATIC CORD LESIONS
Varicocele

A varicocele, consisting of abnormally dilated spermatic cord veins, is the most commonly presenting spermatic cord mass. They are found in 15% of adult men, and may be either idiopathic or secondary.[11] Idiopathic varicoceles are thought to be caused by incompetent valves within the testicular veins and are more common on the left. The course of the left testicular vein is longer, inserting into the left renal vein, and the testicular vein may enlarge as a consequence of compression of the renal vein between the superior mesenteric artery and aorta. These factors combine to increase pressure in the left testicular vein, predisposing to incompetent valves and a varicocele. Further imaging is recommended in the older man with a new onset varicocele because this may be a manifestation of an intra-abdominal mass.[12] Varicoceles are also implicated in infertility, with up to 40% of infertile men being affected. The currently acknowledged link is that varicoceles increase scrotal temperature and adversely affect spermatogenesis, resulting in suboptimal fertility. There is a 30% to 55% reported pregnancy rate for partners of men with infertility postvaricocele ligation.[13] Physical examination reveals a scrotal mass that is described as a "bag of worms." On ultrasonography, a varicocele appears as multiple hypoechoic serpiginous structures posterior to the testis, larger than 2 mm in diameter (**Fig. 5**). Slow venous flow within the varicocele may occasionally produce low-level echoes, but usually no color flow is present at rest. The Valsalva maneuver can be used to confirm the presence of a varicocele, which demonstrates expansion and flow reversal on color Doppler ultrasonography.

Appendix Testis Torsion

An important differential diagnosis to spermatic cord torsion in children is torsion of the appendix testis. Clinically, the pain is localized to the upper pole, and the presence of a tender nodule is suggestive of this diagnosis. Ultrasonographic appearances are of an ovoid mass displaying characteristics similar to that of the epididymis.[14] Appendages are sometimes pedunculated and are at risk of torsion. A torsed appendix testis demonstrates variable reflectivity with increased adjacent color Doppler flow and is associated

with a small surrounding hydrocele (**Fig. 6**). Ultrasonography is a valuable tool in differentiating this condition from testicular torsion, which is a urological emergency.

Lipoma

A lipoma is the most common extratesticular tumor and can occur at any age, with other benign spermatic cord tumors such as leiomyoma, dermoid, and lymphangioma seen less often. A lipoma is often hyperechoic on ultrasonography owing to fat content but can exhibit a varied appearance and may even be hypoechoic (**Fig. 7**). A hernia and malignant sarcoma can also appear hyperechoic, with surgical excision advocated in the absence of a clear diagnosis. Accurate characterization with magnetic resonance (MR) imaging can be performed; a lipoma demonstrates high signal intensity on T1- and T2-weighted sequences and can be differentiated from hemorrhagic lesions on fat-suppressed images. If the MR imaging characteristics do not confirm a lipoma, then the risk of malignancy of the spermatic cord mass increases to 56%.[15] Most malignant spermatic cord tumors are sarcomas and usually present as a scrotal mass. The most frequent scrotal sarcomas are rhabdomyosarcoma, more common in children, and liposarcoma, more common in adults.[16]

EPIDIDYMAL LESIONS
Epididymal Cysts and Spermatoceles

The most common epididymal mass is a cyst, which may be either a true epididymal cyst, being lined by epithelium and containing serous fluid, or a spermatocele (**Fig. 8**), which is secondary to spermatic duct obstruction. About 20% to 40%

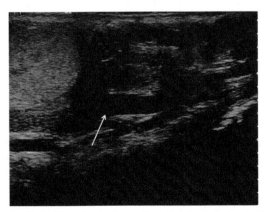

Fig. 5. A dilated vein (*arrow*) at the lower aspect of the left testis, with internal echoes in keeping with a varicocele.

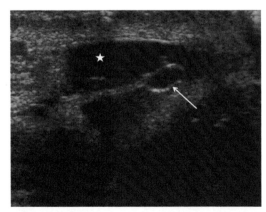

Fig. 6. A long stalk is seen to a cystic appendix testis (*arrow*) with surrounding fluid (*star*) of a small hydrocele in a man with scrotal pain and thought to have a torsion of the appendix testis.

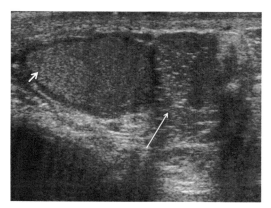

Fig. 7. The testis (*short arrow*) is displaced by an echogenic lesion (*long arrow*): a scrotal lipoma.

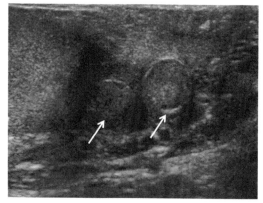

Fig. 9. Two well-circumscribed lesions (*arrows*) in the epididymal tail of medium-level echoes: adenomatoid lesions.

of asymptomatic people are reported to have epididymal cysts, with true epididymal cysts accounting for 75% in the general population.[17] On an ultrasonogram, epididymal cysts and spermatoceles appear as well-circumscribed anechoic lesions demonstrating posterior acoustic enhancement and cannot be differentiated from each other.

Adenomatoid Tumor

Most epididymal tumors are benign, with the most common being an adenomatoid tumor, followed by a lipoma. Most patients are 20 to 50 years of age and present with a painless scrotal lump. On ultrasonography, an adenomatoid tumor (**Fig. 9**) is typically found in the epididymal tail and appears hyperechoic and rounded, with growth of up to 5 cm. Adenomatoid lesions may be found anywhere along the epididymis and the tunica albuginea,

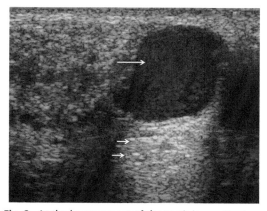

Fig. 8. At the lower aspect of the testis is a cystic structure (*long arrow*) containing debris and demonstrating posterior acoustic enhancement (*short arrows*): a spermatocele.

where they appear to be intratesticular and cannot be distinguished from germ cell tumors.[18]

Papillary Cystadenoma

A papillary cystadenoma is a benign tumor of the epididymis and is associated with von Hippel-Lindau (VHL) disease. Twenty-five percent of patients with VHL have an epididymal papillary cystadenoma, with 40% being bilateral, which is described as pathognomonic for VHL. These tumors are usually solid and echogenic on ultrasonography; however, a cystic appearance may also be seen.[19]

Malignant epididymal tumors are rarely seen and include metastases, sarcomas, and lymphoma.

INTRATESTICULAR LESIONS
Testicular Infarction Following Spermatic Cord Torsion

Torsion of the testis occurs following twisting of the spermatic cord and interruption of the vascular supply to the testis. Spermatic cord torsion classically presents with acute scrotal pain, nausea, and vomiting, commonly followed by ipsilateral scrotal swelling. The prevailing mechanism is believed to be because of a narrow mesenteric pedicle from the spermatic cord with a small testicular bare area (part of the testis not covered by the tunica vaginalis); this enables the testis to rotate within the tunica vaginalis similar to a "bell-clapper."[20] Testicular torsion is clinically important because it culminates in testicular infarction and is reversible if the diagnosis is made early. Testicular infarction begins within 2 hours after vascular occlusion, with irreversible ischemia after 6 hours and established testicular infarction by 24 hours.[21] Eighty-five percent of patients with spermatic cord torsion are between 12 and 18 years of age, with a reported incidence of 1 in 4000 in men younger than 25 years of age, after which, the incidence decreases.[22] The testes enlarge during puberty, increasing in volume by a factor of 5; this enlargement increases the tendency to rotate within the tunica, which explains the higher prevalence of torsion in this age group. In patients with a classic history and examination, surgery is expedited to improve the chances of testicular survival. Spermatic cord torsion must be differentiated from epididymo-orchitis, which is treated conservatively with antibiotics, not surgery, and which can also present in a similar manner.

Testicular torsion begins with the development of venous congestion and subsequent edema of the testis and surrounding structures and is visualized on B-mode as enlargement of the testis with decreased echogenicity. As the ischemia progresses, the testis appears heterogeneous and hypoechoic, in keeping with infarction. In the absence of surgery, hyperechoic areas may occur on a background of infarction, representing hemorrhage.[23] The epididymis becomes progressively larger and more heterogeneous, and it may be possible to identify the twisted spermatic cord, termed the "whirlpool" sign (**Fig. 10**).[24] Color Doppler ultrasonography can be used to differentiate between epididymo-orchitis, in which there is increased vascularity, and torsion, with a reduced or absent blood supply.[25] Vascularity of the testis can be assessed only when compared with the asymptomatic side; therefore, demonstration of color flow in the normal testis is essential to serve as a baseline. This method helps to differentiate torsion from epididymo-orchitis in the adult testis. Absence of color Doppler flow in the pediatric population may be misleading; there is poor sensitivity at detecting color flow linked to the smaller testis. Even with

recent advances in technology, there remains conflicting evidence regarding color flow demonstration in pediatric testes.[26,27] Despite the combination of B-mode with color Doppler ultrasonography, incorrect interpretation of the findings arise, leading to a delay in diagnosis and appropriate intervention. Reasons include the level of experience of the examiner and technical and patient factors. The natural course of spermatic cord torsion is more stepwise; rather than the sudden interruption to vascular flow, swelling impairs venous drainage and results in further edema, which finally culminates in arterial occlusion, adding to clinical uncertainty.[21] Although ultrasonography is a valuable tool in the diagnosis of spermatic cord torsion, it is not infallible and must be used in combination with clinical findings to ensure the best outcome.

Segmental Testicular Infarction

Segmental testicular infarction is a rare condition in which part of the testis infarcts, resulting in acute scrotal pain. Several causative factors have been postulated, including epididymo-orchitis, trauma, sickle cell disease, and previous surgery.[28] The most common cause is infection, which affects an older population more than those with spermatic cord torsion. Segmental testicular infarction demonstrates varying ultrasonographic characteristics: a solitary wedge or round area, mixed or low echogenicity, no anatomic predilection, and reduced or absent color Doppler flow.[28] A significant minority of these lesions exhibit mass effect and may mimic a testicular tumor (**Fig. 11**). In these cases, demonstration of vascularity is critical; flow is increased in malignancy and reduced or absent in infarction. Clinical history and ultrasonographic appearances often enable a confident diagnosis, which helps to avoid

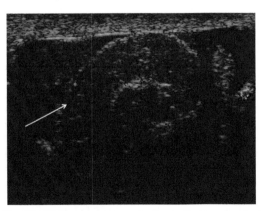

Fig. 10. At the upper aspect of a testis in suspected torsion, the spermatic cord is seen to be twisted (*arrow*) with no color Doppler flow: the 'whirlpool' sign of spermatic cord torsion.

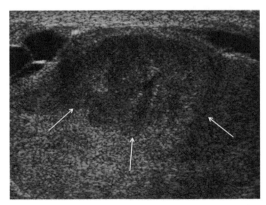

Fig. 11. An irregular focal area (*arrows*) of low reflectivity in the testis is an area of infarction: segmental testicular infarction.

surgery and allow follow-up of this benign condition.

Intratesticular Hematoma

An intratesticular hematoma is an unusual complication of testicular trauma and results in a focal lesion with variable characteristics.[29] Although a positive history is suggestive of the diagnosis, this is not always forthcoming. If imaged acutely a hematoma appears as a well-defined heterogeneous focal lesion with patchy areas of increased reflectivity. Internal echoes may be seen, and no vascularity is demonstrated on color Doppler flow; a hypoechoic rim may occasionally be seen and is believed to be secondary to edema. Intratesticular malignancy is the main differential and is less likely in the presence of a positive history, negative tumor markers, absence of vascularity, and reduction in size on sequential studies. With time, the lesion becomes increasingly hypoechoic and smaller in size before resolving completely.[30]

Intratesticular Varicocele

While extratesticular varicoceles are a common occurrence, their intratesticular counterparts are a rarity, with an incidence of less than 2% in a symptomatic population.[31] Although intra- and extratesticular varicoceles share a common physiologic basis, intratesticular varicoceles are usually found in isolation. Patients commonly present with scrotal pain, the cause of which has been attributed to distension of the tunica albuginea secondary to venous congestion, with a possible association with infertility. An anechoic serpiginous lesion, often with internal echoes, involving the mediastinum testis, with extension into the subcapsular veins has been described.[32] Color Doppler ultrasonography differentiates this type of lesion from other intratesticular cystic lesions, which include rete testis and a simple cyst; vascularity is seen with engorgement and retrograde flow on Valsalva maneuver, similar to that seen in extratesticular varicoceles (**Fig. 12**).

Orchitis

Orchitis often occurs as an element of epididymoorchitis, but primary orchitis without epididymitis can occasionally arise secondary to mumps or human immunodeficiency virus infection.[33] The affected testis initially appears diffusely heterogeneous and hypoechoic, secondary to edema, with sequential examinations demonstrating progression into more focal regions of low reflectivity and an increase in vascularity; illustration of intratesticular venous flow on color Doppler ultrasonography is believed to be characteristic of

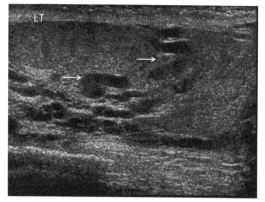

Fig. 12. Serpiginous vessels with internal echoes (*arrows*) course through the testis: intratesticular varicocele.

orchitis.[34,35] With an increase in edema and a reduction in venous return, areas of venous infarction can develop and associated hemorrhage may occur, signified by mixed or high reflectivity. It is important to identify complications, such as abscess formation, infarction, and necrosis. Following treatment, the testicular abnormalities may resolve completely, or result in a loss of volume with fibrosis, giving rise to a heterogeneous parenchyma pattern.

Venous Infarction

Venous infarction may occur with severe epididymoorchitis, whereby edema produces venous impairment and subsequent ischemia (**Fig. 13**). If edema is prolonged, irreversible infarction may affect focal areas of the testis.[36] The testis appears edematous and of heterogeneously low echogenicity; the absence of color Doppler flow with a compatible

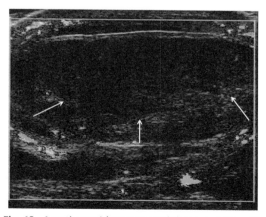

Fig. 13. A patient with severe epididymo-orchitis with persistent pain has an avascular area (*arrows*) in the affected testis: an example of venous infarction.

history is diagnostic.[37] Reversal of arterial flow in the testicular artery during diastole may be present with venous infarction.

Epidermoid Cyst

Epidermoid cysts account for the majority of benign testicular tumors, most commonly seen in men aged 20 to 40 years, and present as a painless scrotal mass.[38] Epidermoid cysts originate from germ cells, contain varying quantities of keratin, and are also known as keratocysts. The quantity, degree of compaction, and maturation of keratin accounts for the ultrasonographic appearances. Four ultrasonographic patterns have been described: (1) type 1 represents the classic "onion-ring" appearance, with alternating layers of high and low reflectivity, corresponding to compacted keratin and loose squamous cells; (2) type 2 appears as a mass with dense calcification and no cyst formation; (3) type 3 is a well-defined cyst with either peripheral or central calcification; and (4) type 4 denotes a mixed pattern, with an ill-defined heterogeneous solid mass.[39] The onion-skin lesion is often described as being pathognomonic (**Fig. 14**). To improve diagnostic confidence, it is important to demonstrate an absence of color Doppler flow with negative tumor markers; the nonspecific features often result in an unnecessary orchidectomy.

Sarcoidosis

Sarcoidosis is a multisystem inflammatory disorder of unknown cause and is characterized by the presence of noncaseating granulomata. Genital involvement is uncommon, with a reported incidence at autopsy of up to 4.5%; however, only 0.5% of these patients were clinically symptomatic.[40] When genital sarcoidosis is suspected, epididymal infiltration is most commonly seen, with isolated intratesticular lesions being infrequent. Testicular sarcoidosis is a diagnosis of exclusion with nonspecific findings on ultrasonography; it appears as a well-defined hypoechoic lesion that may be focal or multifocal and does not demonstrate color Doppler flow. A confident diagnosis can be made if there is clinical evidence of active sarcoidosis and epididymal involvement and if the testicular lesions are multifocal. However, in the absence of these features, histologic diagnosis may be necessary.

Testicular Abscess

A testicular abscess is a rare complication of severe epididymo-orchitis and has also been described following mumps, trauma, and infarction.[41] Ultrasonography demonstrates a focal complex lesion that is heterogeneous and hypoechoic with shaggy irregular margins. No vascularity is seen on color Doppler flow, and internal echoes may be evident (**Fig. 15**). If the clinical history is in keeping with an abscess, orchidectomy is the treatment of choice.

Testicular Adrenal Rest Tumors

Congenital adrenal hyperplasia (CAH) is an inherited disorder of impaired adrenal steroid synthesis, characterized by 21α-hydroxylase enzyme deficiency in more than 90% of cases. Testicular adrenal rest tumors are benign intratesticular lesions that are associated with CAH and believed to arise from aberrant adrenal tissue that descends with the testes during development. Although previously thought to be uncommon, recent reports have demonstrated a high prevalence of these tumors in patients with CAH, up to 94% in one series.[42] Most of these tumors are seen in the presence of known CAH; however, they may present as the first manifestation of

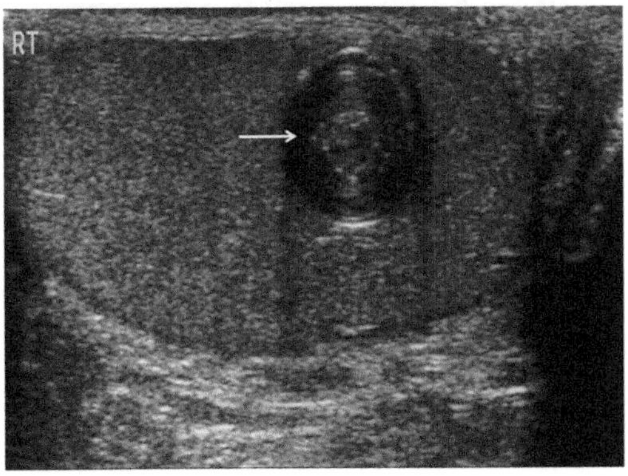

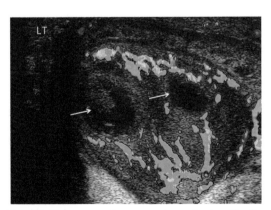

Fig. 14. A well-circumscribed intratesticular lesion with the classical onion-ring appearance (*arrow*) of an epidermoid cyst.

Fig. 15. Two separate, avascular mixed reflective lesions (*arrows*) in a patient with severe epididymo-orchitis: intratesticular abscesses.

CAH. Clinically, the significance lies in the association with infertility, secondary to direct compression of the seminiferous tubules or by local steroid effects on the Leydig cells. On ultrasonography, the lesions appear as lobulated hypoechoic foci that occur near the mediastinum testis, with little distortion to the testicular structure, and exhibit fibrosis, with acoustic shadowing (**Fig. 16**). Color Doppler ultrasonography reveals no change in the underlying vascular pattern, and a "spoke-wheel" pattern of increased vascularity has been reported in most tumors.[43]

Intratesticular Tumors

Approximately 1% of all malignancies in men are testicular in origin; these tumors are the most common in the 15- to 34-year-old age group. In 2009, an estimated 8400 new cases were diagnosed, and 380 men died of testicular cancer, with the 5-year survival rate currently predicted at 95.3%. These high survival rates are in part due to tumor sensitivity to chemotherapy and radiotherapy and also to the early patient appreciation of an abnormality in a superficial organ.[44] Early diagnosis is crucial, and ultrasonography is the gold standard imaging modality. Even original ultrasonography alone has high sensitivity. Risk factors for testicular cancer include a past history of testicular carcinoma, cryptorchidism, infertility, and Klinefelter syndrome.[45] The most common presentation is of a painless scrotal mass, with pain being reported in only 10%. Once an intratesticular lesion is demonstrated, the B-mode appearance and presence of vascularity on color Doppler ultrasonography are often used to differentiate between benign and malignant disease. This is especially important because of the diversity of benign testicular lesions that mimic the appearances of testicular cancer, such as

infarction, hematoma, sarcoidosis, and epidermoid cysts.

GERM CELL TUMORS

Germ cell tumors account for 95% of testicular malignancies and can be divided into seminomatous and nonseminomatous groups; the remainder are made up of sex cord stromal tumors, lymphoma, and metastases. The seminomatous tumors are the most common pure germ cell tumor and comprise up to 50% of all germ cell tumors. If nonseminomatous elements are discovered within the mass, then management follows the nonseminomatous route.

Seminoma

A seminoma occurs in an older population with an average age of 40 years. Disease is limited to the testis in 70%, with retroperitoneal spread in 20% and extranodal metastases in 5%; bilateral disease is rare, occurring in only 2%.[45] Elevated β-human chorionic gonadotrophic hormone levels have been reported in 83% of patients, and α-fetoprotein (AFP) is never elevated; if an increased level of AFP is discovered, the tumor is treated as nonseminomatous.[46] At histology, a seminoma may vary in size from small well-defined lesions to masses that completely replace normal testicular parenchyma; the cells are comparatively uniform with clear cytoplasm and lymphoid infiltrate. This uniformity seen in a seminoma is also found on ultrasonography; the lesions are typically hypoechoic and homogeneous, with cystic areas found in 10% (**Fig. 17**).[47]

Nonseminomatous Germ Cell Tumors

Nonseminomatous germ cell tumors of the mixed type are more common than those containing

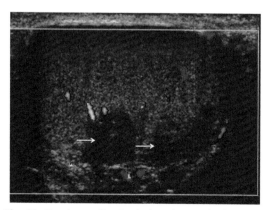

Fig. 16. Two low-reflective lesions (*arrows*) of adrenal rest cells. (*Courtesy of* W.K. Chong, MD, Chapel Hill, NC).

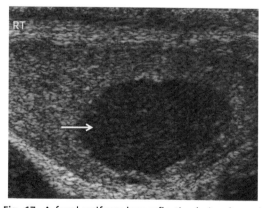

Fig. 17. A focal uniform low-reflective lesion (*arrow*) demonstrating classic features of a seminoma.

pure cell lines, accounting for 32% to 60% of all germ cell tumors, with embryonal cell carcinoma being the most frequent constituent.[48] Common patterns include (1) teratoma, embryonal cell carcinoma, yolk sac tumor, and hormone-containing syncytiotrophoblast; (2) teratoma and embryonal cell carcinoma; and (3) seminoma and embryonal cell carcinoma, although any combination can be found. The ultrasonographic findings reflect the diversity of the components and characteristically appear irregular with a heterogeneous parenchyma pattern. Echogenic foci, representing calcification, hemorrhage, or fibrosis, are found in 35%, and cystic components in 61% (**Fig. 18**).[47,48]

EMBRYONAL CELL CARCINOMA

Pure embryonal cell carcinoma makes up 2% to 3% of all germ cell tumors. An embryonal cell carcinoma is an aggressive tumor with ultrasonographic findings often demonstrating irregular and indistinct margins, with a heterogeneous echo texture. These tumors are characteristically smaller in size than a seminoma without enlargement of the testis, although invasion of the tunica albuginea may occur resulting in distortion of the testicular outline.

YOLK SAC TUMOR

Yolk sac tumors are also known as endodermal sinus tumors, most of which occur in children younger than 2 years.[49] Elevated AFP levels are found in 90% of yolk sac tumors, as AFP is normally produced by the embryonic yolk sac and can be used to monitor treatment response. B-mode appearances are nonspecific and can range from being diffusely heterogeneous to testicular enlargement without a focal mass, which is found in the pediatric population. Although the presence of yolk sac components usually indicates poor prognosis, outcomes can be excellent when disease is limited to the testis, as it is in more than 80% of patients.

TERATOMA

A teratoma is the second most common pediatric testicular tumor, and a mature teratoma is often benign in children. In adults, a pure teratoma is rare and the majority of these tumors occurr as part of a mixed germ cell tumor. But, as opposed to children, they must all be considered malignant. All 3 germ cell layers (endoderm, mesoderm, and ectoderm) are found in a disorganized arrangement within a teratoma.[48] The imaging findings mirror the complex nature of the tumor, and they typically appear as large, well-circumscribed, heterogeneous masses with echogenic foci that may represent calcification, cartilage, immature bone, or fibrosis. Cyst formation is more common than in other germ cell tumors, their appearance being dependent on the contents of the cyst, with serous fluid in anechoic simple cysts or mucoid/keratinous fluid in complex cysts (see **Fig. 18**).

CHORIOCARCINOMA

Choriocarcinoma is a rare and highly aggressive germ cell tumor. In its pure form, it is seen in only 0.3% of cases, but microscopic foci are demonstrable in 16% of mixed germ cell tumors. Choriocarcinoma carries the worst prognosis of all germ cell tumors, with early metastatic spread to the lung, liver, gastrointestinal tract, and brain, and is associated with an elevated human chorionic gonadotropin level. On ultrasonography, choriocarcinoma is seen as focal masses with solid and cystic components; the cystic elements represent hemorrhagic necrosis.

Sex Cord Stromal Tumors

Sex cord stromal tumors account for 4% of all testicular malignancies; they originate from the Sertoli cells that form the sex cords and the Leydig cells of the interstitium. Sex cord stromal tumors are characteristically small in size, and most of these tumors are discovered incidentally. The B-mode appearances are of a well-circumscribed, homogeneous, hypoechoic lesion, and although 90% of these tumors are benign, there are no specific imaging features to determine malignant potential. As a result, all of these lesions are resected.

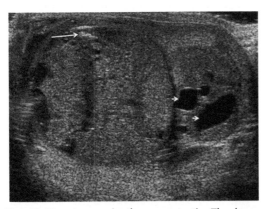

Fig. 18. Two tumors in the same testis. The larger tumor, a teratoma, demonstrates a focal area of calcification (*long arrow*), while the smaller mixed germ cell tumor demonstrates pockets of cystic change (*short arrows*).

LEYDIG CELL TUMORS

Leydig cell tumors comprise most of the sex cord stromal tumors and can be found in all age groups. Androgens or estrogens may be secreted by Leydig cell tumors, giving rise to symptoms such as gynecomastia, decreased libido, and precocious virilization in approximately 30% of patients, with a further 43% of cases presenting with scrotal swelling. Most tumors appear as a small hypoechoic mass on ultrasonography, but cyst formation, hemorrhage, and necrosis have all been described (**Fig. 19**).[50]

SERTOLI CELL TUMORS

Sertoli cell tumors contribute only 1% to testicular malignancies and have varied appearances ranging from well-circumscribed focal lobulated masses to diffuse parenchyma heterogeneity.[51] Large cell calcifying Sertoli cell tumor is a subtype that, as the name suggests, demonstrates multiple areas of calcification on ultrasonography and is associated with Peutz-Jeghers and Carney syndrome.

Testicular Lymphoma and Leukemia

Testicular lymphoma is seen in less than 1% of patients with systemic lymphoma and represents 5% of all testicular malignancies. Testicular lymphoma is the most common testicular malignancy in men older than 60 years, and these tumors are almost all B-cell lymphomas. Ultrasonographic findings are variable but usually consist of focal or multifocal hypoechoic lesions that may infiltrate the entire testicle.[52] Although primary leukemia of the testes is a rare occurrence, secondary involvement is more common, with up to 65% of acute leukemia cases and 20% to 35% of chronic leukemia cases demonstrating testicular infiltration at autopsy. Ultrasonographic appearances are similar to those of lymphoma and are indistinguishable from germ cell tumors (**Fig. 20**). Metastatic testicular disease is rare and is most commonly described in primary prostatic and lung cancer.

TESTICULAR CALCIFICATION

Testicular microlithiasis is characterized by microcalcification within the testis. An accepted categorization is into classical testicular microlithiasis (the presence of 5 or more echogenic foci within the testis on a single ultrasonographic view) and limited testicular microlithiasis (<5 microliths per ultrasonographic field).[53,54] The calcified foci measure only 1 to 3 mm in diameter, and the majority do not demonstrate acoustic shadowing, which is an important distinguishing feature from other forms of intratesticular calcification. The ultrasonographic appearances are typically random and symmetric, although asymmetry and clustering are often seen. There is controversy with regard to the association of testicular microlithiasis with primary testicular tumors; an increase of prevalence is established, but the incidence is unknown.[54] Opinions regarding the management pathway of patients with testicular microlithiasis are divided, but given the association with testicular malignancy, regular surveillance has been advocated either with ultrasonography or physical examination.[55] There is also an association of macrocalcification with primary testicular tumors, and surveillance of these patients is also suggested.[56] Calcification is thought to be related to the concept of the "burned out" germ cell tumor and the phenomenon of primary tumor regression (**Fig. 21**). The suspected

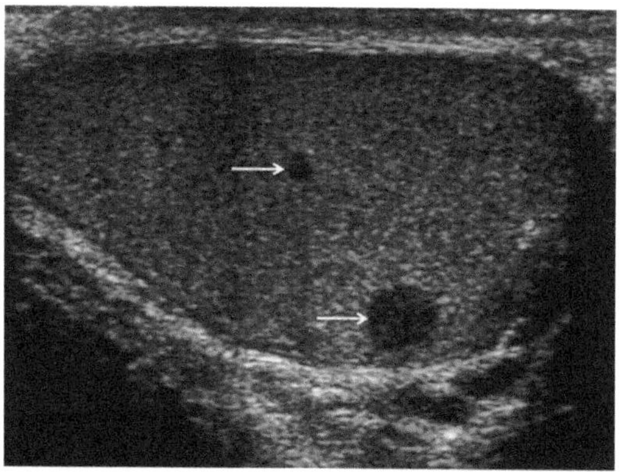

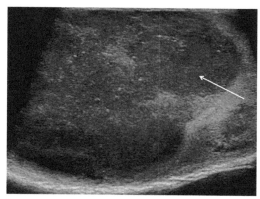

Fig. 19. Two small low-reflective lesions (*arrows*), which were Leydig cell tumors on histology.

Fig. 20. The testis is largely replaced by a mixed-reflective lesion (*arrow*) found to be lymphoma.

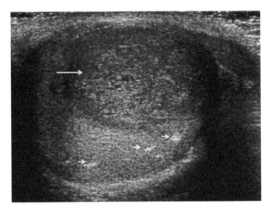

Fig. 21. A mixed germ cell tumor (*long arrow*) in a testis with areas of macrocalcification (*short arrows*) outside the tumor, raising the possibility of areas of burnt-out tumor.

mechanism is of a rapidly growing germ cell tumor, usually teratocarcinoma or choriocarcinoma, outgrowing its blood supply and subsequently collapsing on itself; histology frequently demonstrates few or no tumor cells. Focal areas of macrocalcification are often found in patients with metastatic germ cell tumor, during a search for the primary.[57]

NORMAL VARIANTS
Two-Tone Testis

"Two-tone testis" describes the appearance of 2 parts of the testis that have been transected by a normal variant, the transmediastinal vessels; the parenchyma nearest the probe is of normal reflectivity, whereas the segment on the distal side of the vessels is of reduced/low reflectivity.[58] This unusual appearance is thought to result from refractive artifact produced by oblique imaging through the transmediastinal vessels (**Fig. 22**).

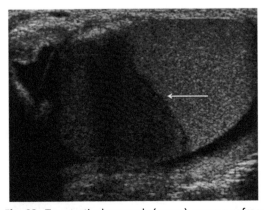

Fig. 22. Transtesticular vessels (*arrow*) cause a refractive artifact and result in the two-tone testis appearance.

Polyorchidism

Polyorchidism is a rare abnormality defined as the existence of more than 2 testes, with 3 testes being most common. It is classified into 4 types: (1) type A, a supernumerary testis without either the epididymis or vas deferens; (2) type B, a supernumerary testis and epididymis but no vas deferens; (3) type C, a supernumerary testis with a separate epididymis and sharing of the vas deferens with the ipsilateral testis; (4) type D, a supernumerary testis with an entirely independent epididymis and vas deferens.[5]

Rete Testis

Dilatation of the rete testis is common, occurs mostly in patients older than 50 years, and is normally either postinfectious or posttraumatic.[59] B-mode imaging reveals multiple hypoechoic ovoid structures within, or adjacent to, the mediastinum testis. The cysts are typically only a few millimeters in size, do not demonstrate vascular flow on color Doppler ultrasonography, and are bilateral in up to a third of patients. In patients with azoospermia, the finding of rete testis distension is significant because it implies ipsilateral spermatic duct obstruction. Furthermore, it is important to exclude an intratesticular tumor because a dilated rete testis has been described in association with a seminoma, teratoma, and an epididymal cystadenoma.[60]

REFERENCES

1. Satchithananda K, Aziz ZA, Sidhu PS. Pelvis male genital tract. In: Sidhu PS, Chong WK, editors. Measurement in ultrasound. A practical handbook. 1st edition. London: Arnold; 2004. p. 95–132.
2. Levenson RB, Singh AK, Novelline RA. Fournier gangrene: role of imaging. Radiographics 2008;28: 519–28.
3. Rajan DK, Scharer A. Radiology of Fournier's gangrene. AJR Am J Roentgenol 1998;170:163–8.
4. Dogra VS, Gottlieb RH, Oka M, et al. Sonography of the scrotum. Radiology 2003;227:18–36.
5. Stewart VR, Sidhu PS. The testis: the unusual, the rare and the bizarre. Clin Radiol 2007;62: 289–302.
6. Leung ML, Gooding GA, Williams RD. High-resolution sonography of scrotal contents in asymptomatic subjects. AJR Am J Roentgenol 1984;143:161–4.
7. Ogata M, Imai S, Hosotani R, et al. Abdominal ultrasonography for the diagnosis of strangulation in small bowel obstruction. Br J Surg 1994;81: 421–4.

8. Freeman JL, Jafri SZ, Roberts JL, et al. CT of congenital and aquired abnormalities of the spleen. Radiographics 1993;13:597–610.

9. Stewart VR, Sellars ME, Somers S, et al. Splenogonadal fusion: B-Mode and color Doppler sonographic appearances. J Ultrasound Med 2004;23:1087–90.

10. Guarin U, Dimitrieva Z, Ashley SJ. Splenogonald fusion. A rare congenital anomaly demonstrated by 99mTc-sulfur colloid imaging: case report. J Nucl Med 1975;16:922–4.

11. Meacham RB, Townsend RR, Rademacher D, et al. The incidence of varicoceles in the general population when evaluated by physical examination, gray scale sonography and color Doppler sonography. J Urol 1994;151:1535–8.

12. El-Saeity NS, Sidhu PS. "Scrotal varicocele, exclude a renal tumour". Is this evidence based? Clin Radiol 2006;61:593–9.

13. Kim ED, Lipshultz LI. Role of ultrasound in the assessment of male infertility. J Clin Ultrasound 1996;24:437–53.

14. Sellars ME, Sidhu PS. Ultrasound appearances of the testicular appendages: pictorial review. Eur Radiol 2003;13:127–35.

15. Beccia DJ, Krane RJ, Olsson CA. Clinical management of non-testicular intrascrotal tumors. J Urol 1976;116:476–9.

16. Woodward PJ, Schwab CM, Sesterhenn IA. Extra-testicular scrotal masses: radiologic-pathologic correlation. Radiographics 2003;23:215–40.

17. Holden A, List A. Extra-testicular lesions: a radiological and pathological correlation. Australas Radiol 1994;38:99–105.

18. Somers WJ. The sonographic appearance of an intratesticular adenomatoid tumor. J Clin Ultrasound 1992;20:479–80.

19. Alexander JA, Lichtman JB, Varma JB. Ultrasound demonstration of a papillary cystadenoma of the epididymis. J Clin Ultrasound 1991;19:442–5.

20. Corriere JN. Horizontal lie of the testicle: a diagnostic sign and torsion of the testis. J Urol 1972;107:616–7.

21. Sidhu PS. Clinical and imaging features of testicular torsion: role of ultrasound. Clin Radiol 1999; 54:343–52.

22. Williamson RCN. Torsion of the testis and allied conditions. Br J Surg 1976;63:465–76.

23. Bird K, Rosenfield AT, Taylor KJ. Ultrasonography in testicular torsion. Radiology 1983;147:527–34.

24. Vijayaraghavan SB. Sonographic differential diagnosis of acute scrotum: real-time whirlpool sign, a key sign of torsion. J Ultrasound Med 2006;25: 563–74.

25. Lerner RG, Mevorach RA, Hulbert WC, et al. Color Doppler US in the evaluation of acute scrotal disease. Radiology 1990;176:355–8.

26. Atkinson GO, Patrick LE, Ball TI, et al. The normal and abnormal scrotum in children: evaluation with color Doppler sonography. Am J Roentgenol 1992; 158:613–7.

27. Albrecht T, Lotzof K, Hussain HK, et al. Power Doppler US of the normal prepubertal testis: does it live up to its promises? Radiology 1997;203:227–31.

28. Bilagi P, Sriprasad S, Clarke JL, et al. Clinical and ultrasound features of segmental testicular infarction: six-year experience from a single centre. Eur Radiol 2007;17:2810–8.

29. Purushothaman H, Sellars ME, Clarke JL, et al. Intratesticular haematoma: differentiation from tumour on clinical history and ultrasound appearances in two cases. Br J Radiol 2007;80:e184–7.

30. Megremis S, Michalakou M, Mattheakis M, et al. An unusual well-circumscribed intratesticular traumatic hematoma: diagnosis and follow-up by sonography. J Ultrasound Med 2005;24:547–50.

31. Browne RF, Geoghegan T, Torreggiani WC. Intratesticular varicocele. Australas Radiol 2005;49:333–4.

32. Atasoy C, Fitoz S. Gray-scale and color Doppler sonographic findings in intratesticular varicocele. J Clin Ultrasound 2001;29:369–73.

33. Dogra VS, Bhatt S. Acute painful scrotum. Radiol Clin North Am 2004;42:349–63.

34. Cook JL, Dewbury K. The changes seen on high-resolution ultrasound in orchitis. Clin Radiol 2000; 55:13–8.

35. Horstman WG, Middleton WD, Melson GL. Scrotal inflammatory disease: color Doppler US findings. Radiology 1991;179:55–9.

36. Bird K, Rosenfield AT. Testicular infarction secondary to acute inflammatory disease: demonstration by B-scan ultrasound. Radiology 1984;152:785–8.

37. Eisner DJ, Goldman SM, Petronis J, et al. Bilateral testicular infarction caused by epididymitis. AJR Am J Roentgenol 1991;157:517–9.

38. Shah KH, Maxted WC, Chun B. Epidermoid cysts of the testis: a report of three cases and an analysis of 141 cases from the world literature. Cancer 1981;47:577–82.

39. Atchley JT, Dewbury KC. Ultrasound appearances of testicular epidermoid cysts. Clin Radiol 2000;55: 493–502.

40. Ricker W, Clarke M. Sarcoidosis: a clinicopathological review of 300 cases including 22 autopsies. Am J Clin Pathol 1949;19:725.

41. Dogra VS, Gottlieb RH, Rubens DJ, et al. Benign intratesticular cystic lesions: US features. Radiographics 2001;21:S273–81.

42. Stikkelbroeck NM, Otten BJ, Pasic A, et al. High prevalance of testicular adrenal rest tumors, impaired spermatogenesis and Leydig cell failure in adolescent and adult males with congenital adrenal hyperplasia. J Clin Endocrinol Metab 2001;86:5721–8.

43. Avila NA, Premkumar A, Shawker TH, et al. Testicular adrenal rest tissue in congenital adrenal hyperplasia: findings at gray-scale and color Doppler US. Radiology 1996;198:99–104.

44. Available at: http://www.seer.cancer.gov/csr/1975_2006/results_single/sect_01_table.01.pdf. Accessed March 19, 2010.

45. Horwich A, Shipley J, Huddart RA. Testicular germ cell cancer. Lancet 2006;367:754–65.

46. Javadpour N, McIntire KR, Waldmann TA. Human chorionic gonadotropin (HCG) and alpha-fetoprotein (AFP) in sera and tumor cells of patients with testicular seminoma: a prospective study. Cancer 1978;42:2768–72.

47. Schwerk WB, Schwerk WN, Rodeck G. Testicular tumours: prospective analysis of real-time US patterns and abdominal staging. Radiology 1987; 164:369–74.

48. Woodward PJ, Sohaey R, O'Donoghue MJ, et al. Tumors and tumor-like lesions of the testis: radiologic-pathologic correlation. Radiographics 2002;22:189–216.

49. Frush DP, Sheldon CA. Diagnostic imaging for pediatric scrotal disorders. Radiographics 1998; 18:969–85.

50. Kim I, Young RH, Scully RE. Leydig cell tumors of the testis: a clinicopathological analysis of 40 cases and review of the literature. Am J Surg Pathol 1985;9: 177–92.

51. Lui P, Thorner P. Sonographic appearance of Sertoli cell tumor with pathologic correlation. Pediatr Radiol 1993;23:127–8.

52. Mazzu D, Jeffrey RB, Ralls PW. Lymphoma and leukemia involving the testicles: findings on gray-scale and color Doppler sonography. AJR Am J Roentgenol 1995;164:645–7.

53. Backus ML, Mack LA, Middleton WD, et al. Testicular microlithiasis: imaging appearances and pathologic correlation. Radiology 1994;192:781–5.

54. Miller FN, Sidhu PS. Does testicular microlithiasis matter? A review. Clin Radiol 2002;57:883–90.

55. Rashid HH, Cos LR, Weinberg E, et al. Testicular microlithiasis: a review and its association with testicular cancer. Urol Oncol 2004;22:285–9.

56. Miller FN, Rosairo S, Clarke JL, et al. Testicular calcification and microlithiasis: association with primary intra-testicular malignancy in 3,477 patients. Eur Radiol 2006;17:363–9.

57. Comiter CV, Renshaw AA, Benson CB, et al. Burned-out primary testicular cancer: sonographic and pathological characteristics. J Urol 1996;156:85–8.

58. Bushby LH, Sellars ME, Sidhu PS. The "two-tone" testis: spectrum of ultrasound appearances. Clin Radiol 2007;62:1119–23.

59. Sellars ME, Sidhu PS. Pictorial review: ultrasound appearances of the rete testis. Eur J Ultrasound 2001;14:115–20.

60. Hamm B, Fobbe F, Loy V. Testicular cysts: differentiation with US and clinical findings. Radiology 1988; 168:19–23.

Ultrasonography of the Urinary Bladder

Ravinder Sidhu, MD*, Shweta Bhatt, MD,
Vikram S. Dogra, MD

KEYWORDS

- Ultrasonography • Urinary bladder • Distension
- Bladder abnormalities

The urinary bladder is an ideal organ for sonographic examination because of the excellent acoustic properties of fluid (urine) and the superficial location of the urinary bladder. Ultrasound is able to give information about the capacity of the bladder; changes in bladder wall thickness and structure; intraluminal abnormalities such as a mass, a polyp, calculi, hemorrhage, foreign bodies; and also about extrinsic mass lesions that may compress and distort the bladder wall.

ULTRASOUND TECHNIQUE

The patient should have a moderately distended bladder for accurate evaluation of wall thickness, mucosal details, and also for evaluation of the bladder neck and proximal urethra. If the bladder is not sufficiently distended, distension may be obtained by administering saline through a urinary catheter. A high-frequency transducer of 6 to 7 MHz should be used for assessment of the bladder wall. A lower-frequency transducer is used for evaluation of adjacent structures. The patient is typically placed in a dorsal recumbent position. Both sagittal and transverse views should be obtained.

NORMAL SONOGRAPHIC APPEARANCE

A well-distended bladder is seen as an anechoic structure (**Fig. 1**). The shape is usually ovoid to oblong. The 4 anatomic layers of the bladder (the mucosa, the submucosa, the muscular layer, and the serosal layer) are difficult to evaluate separately. However, generally it is possible to distinguish 2 thin, parallel, hyperechoic lines (outer line as serosa/perivascular fat interface) separated by a hypoechoic line (muscularis layer), and another hyperechoic line (lamina propria submucosa paralleling mucosal interface). The normal thickness of the bladder wall varies from 1 to 3 mm in a moderately distended bladder. The thickness should be uniform. The ureteral orifices can be seen as small elevations of mucosa located on either side of the midline at the trigone region (**Fig. 2**). Ureteral jets may be seen intermittently as bright echoes, also called ureteral jet effect (**Fig. 3**). Various theories have been proposed for the appearance of the ureteral jets, including (1) temperature or density difference between ureteral and bladder urine, and (2) microbubble of particulate matter in urine causing turbulence and cavitation at the ureteral orifice.

BLADDER ABNORMALITIES

Pathologic processes in the urinary bladder include both benign and malignant lesions. The common benign entities include calculi, cystitis, bladder hernias, neurogenic bladder, ureterocele, rupture of urinary bladder, fistulas, foreign bodies, and other rare entities such as bladder endometriosis and pseudotumors. The malignant processes include urothelial carcinoma, adenocarcinoma, squamous cell carcinoma, lymphoma, and metastases.

Department of Radiology, University of Rochester Medical Center, 601 Elmwood Avenue, Rochester, NY 14642, USA
* Corresponding author.
E-mail address: ravinder_sidhu@urmc.rochester.edu

Ultrasound Clin 5 (2010) 457–474
doi:10.1016/j.cult.2010.08.001
1556-858X/10/$ — see front matter. Published by Elsevier Inc.

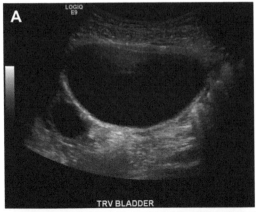

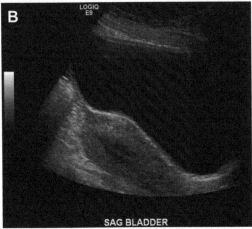

Fig. 1. Normal bladder. Sagittal (*A*) and transverse (*B*) gray-scale ultrasound images of a normal distended bladder.

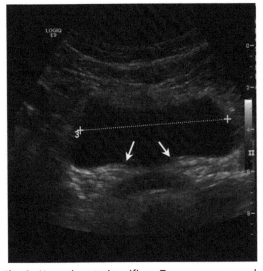

Fig. 2. Normal ureteric orifices. Transverse gray-scale image of the bladder shows the location of the ureteric orifices (*arrows*).

BENIGN LESIONS
Bladder Lithiasis

Both radiopaque and radiolucent calculi can be detected with ultrasound. They are seen as focal, dependent, hyperechoic, curvilinear echogenic foci with acoustic shadowing that usually move with changes in the patient's position unless the stones are very large (**Fig. 4**). However, not all stones show acoustic shadowing. The degree of shadowing correlates with chemical composition, the location of the calculus with respect to the focal zone, and the frequency of the transducer. The false-negative examinations can be caused by inadequate distention of the bladder or the calculus being too small to resolve.

Calculi at the distal ureters or at the ureterovesicle junction can also be detected while evaluating the bladder. Absence of the ureteral jet on one side may suggest obstruction to the ureter (**Fig. 5**).

CYSTITIS

Bladder cystitis is defined as inflammation of the urinary bladder from any cause (**Box 1**). It is a common condition affecting both sexes and seen at all ages, although it is more common in women because of the shortness of the female urethra and also because of the close proximity of the urethra and anus.[1]

Acute and Chronic Cystitis

Cystitis can occur in acute and chronic forms. Acute cystitis is more common than the chronic form. In male patients, the acute form is generally associated with an underlying disorder; hence, male patients with acute cystitis must be thoroughly investigated. In female patients, isolated episodes of cystitis may usually be treated with antibiotics, but repeated episodes require further investigations to rule out associated anatomic abnormality that may be predisposing to the infection.

Chemical Cystitis

Chemical cystitis occurs in the absence of microorganisms. The causative chemicals may include deodorants sprayed in the perineal area, the use of detergents in water, or may be associated with excessive use of wipes. The most important cause that is encountered in clinical practice is the use of cytotoxic drugs, especially the chemotherapeutic agent cyclophosphamide. Cyclophosphamide releases an oxidizing metabolite, acrolein, which causes sloughing of urothelial cells resulting in hemorrhagic cystitis.[2]

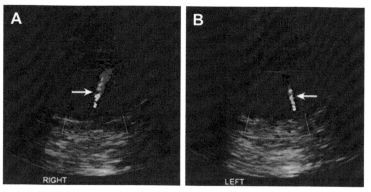

Fig. 3. Normal ureteric jets. Transverse color Doppler images of the bladder (*A, B*) show the appearance of bilateral ureteric jets (*arrows*).

Tubercular Cystitis

Tubercular cystitis is more common in developing countries, but the incidence is increasing in the United States and Europe. Tubercular cystitis is usually secondary to renal tuberculosis. The diagnosis may be difficult because of nonspecific symptoms, clinical results, and imaging findings. Tuberculosis should be considered in patients with refractory cystitis, with sterile pyuria, or patients who originate from countries where tuberculosis is endemic. Patients with immune-compromised

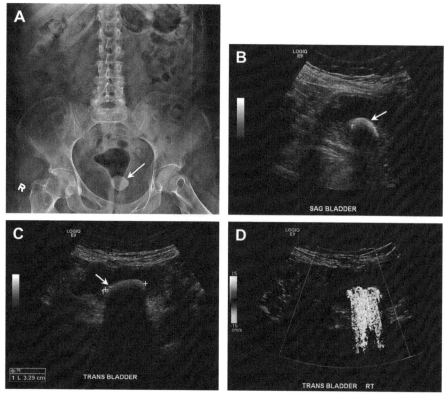

Fig. 4. Bladder calculus. Plain radiograph (*A*) of the abdomen shows a large calcified structure in the pelvis (*arrow*) in the expected location of the bladder. Sagittal (*B*) and transverse (*C*) gray-scale ultrasound images of the bladder show a large calculus within the bladder (*arrow*) with posterior acoustic shadowing. Corresponding color Doppler image (*D*) of the bladder shows twinkle artifact posterior to the calculus.

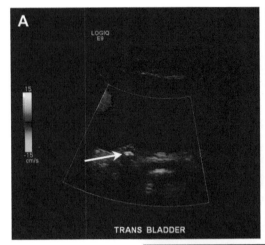
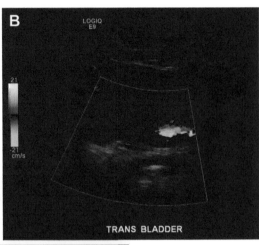
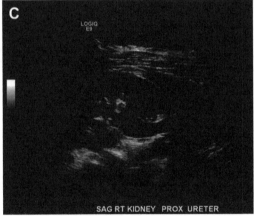

Fig. 5. Obstructing calculus at the ureterovesicle junction. Transverse color Doppler images of the bladder (*A, B*) show a 0.8-cm calculus (*arrow*) at the right ureterovesicle junction, with absence of ureteric jet on that side (*B*). Corresponding sagittal gray-scale ultrasound image (*C*) of the right kidney shows mild to moderate hydronephrosis and hydroureter.

status caused by acquired immunodeficiency syndrome, or organ transplant recipients, are also at higher risk. At cystoscopy, early features of bladder tuberculosis are inflamed bladder wall with a thick, chalky, white, and edematous mucosa. In early tuberculosis, the changes are seen around the ureteric orifices and the trigone of the bladder.[3] Later, fibrosis leads to contracted, small-sized bladder.

Box 1
Types of cystitis
Acute cystitis
Chronic cystitis
Chemical cystitis
Tubercular cystitis
Radiation and chemotherapy cystitis
Interstitial cystitis
Emphysematous cystitis
Schistosomiasis cystitis
Cystitis glandularis

Schistosomiasis Cystitis

Schistosomiasis is the infection caused by *Schistosoma heamatobium*. Schistosomiasis is common in Africa, the Middle East, and the Nile valley. Humans are the definitive host. The embryos penetrate the skin of the host from infected water, migrate to the visceral venous plexus where eggs are laid in the submucosal veins, and penetrate the bladder wall to enter the urine. The eggs cause an inflammatory reaction leading to chronic inflammation, bladder fibrosis, urethral stricture, leukoplakia, squamous metaplasia, and also carcinoma in situ.[4] Imaging findings reflect the pathologic changes.

In the acute phase, nodular bladder wall thickening is seen. There may be ureteral dilatation. The chronic phase is characterized by a contracted, fibrotic, thick-walled bladder with calcifications. The calcifications are typically curvilinear and represent large numbers of calcified eggs within the bladder wall. Calcification may also extend into the distal ureter. Rarely, a mass may develop secondary to inflammation or complicating carcinoma, typically squamous carcinoma.[5] Treatment is medical in the form of praziquantel, which destroys the adult worms and incites the eggs to hatch. However, it has no effect on the chronic fibrotic changes in the bladder wall and ureters.

Radiation and Chemotherapy Cystitis

Severe hemorrhagic cystitis may develop after chemotherapy or irradiation of the bladder. Chemotherapy-induced cystitis occurs from systemic or local chemotherapy. Radiation injury is caused by external radiation, interstitial or intracavity radiation therapy for bladder or other pelvic malignancy in adjoining pelvic organs. The earliest changes are vasodilatation and edema of the bladder wall leading to hemorrhagic cystitis caused by denudation of the urothelium. Late sequelae include ulceration, bladder fibrosis, bladder necrosis, fistula formation, and incontinence. Superimposed secondary bacterial infection may complicate the inflammation.[6] At imaging, there is abnormal bladder wall thickening with focal or diffuse irregular thickening, spasticity, and decreased distensibility (**Fig. 6**).

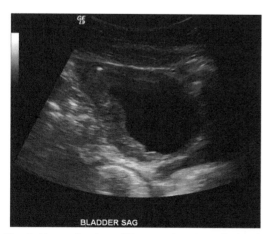

Fig. 6. Hemorrhagic cystitis secondary to radiation in a patient with known metastatic nephroblastoma. Sagittal gray-scale ultrasound image of the bladder in this patient presenting with hematuria shows a thick-walled spastic bladder.

Rarely, calcification can be seen. Gas within the bladder indicates fistula formation unless some procedure has been carried out recently. Treatment is supportive, with blood transfusions and bladder irrigation with instillation of various agents such as alum, silver nitrate, and formalin. Urinary tract diversion or cystectomy may be performed in patients with intractable symptoms.

Interstitial Cystitis

Interstitial cystitis is a chronic submucosal inflammatory disease characterized by chronic urinary urgency, frequency, and pain without evidence of bacterial infection. This condition is predominantly seen in women. Bladder capacity is reduced because of chronic inflammation and fibrosis of the urinary bladder wall.[7]

Emphysematous Cystitis

Emphysematous cystitis is caused by gas-forming bacteria such as *Escherichia coli*. The gas is seen as hyperechoic foci that can be intramural as well as intraluminal in location.[8]

Cystitis Cystica and Cystitis Glandularis

Cystitis cystica and cystitis glandularis are common inflammatory reactive disorders that occur as sequelae of chronic irritation. Metaplasia is caused by calculus, infection, chronic bladder outlet obstruction, and tumor. The urothelium then proliferates into buds that grow down into connective tissue beneath the epithelium in the lamina propria. These buds then differentiate into cystic deposits of cystitis cystica or into intestinal columnar mucin-secreting glands, resulting in cystitis glandularis.[9,10] The histologic features of both cystitis cystica and cystitis glandularis are usually present, rather than either in its pure form. Cystitis glandularis also occurs in association with pelvic lipomatosis and is believed to result from bladder obstruction and chronic infection. Cystitis glandularis and cystitis cystica can occur at any age, and there is a reported prevalence of 2.4% in children with urinary tract infections.[11] A slight male predominance is reported. Symptoms are those of chronic irritation, such as frequency, dysuria, urgency, and hematuria. In rare cases, mucus may be secreted in the urine. At cystoscopy, the mucosa usually has a cobblestone appearance. Cystitis glandularis may develop into a papillary or polypoid mass, a form that mimics carcinoma, with a predilection for the bladder neck and trigone. In young patients, their age should raise the suspicion that the lesion might be nonneoplastic, but biopsy is necessary for a definitive diagnosis. At imaging, the masses from cystitis cystica and cystitis glandularis vary in number and size and are seen as filling defects at urography. On computed tomography (CT) and magnetic resonance (MR) imaging, they may appear as enhancing polypoid masses with variable MR signal intensity. The role of ultrasonography is limited in the diagnosis of these lesions.

The sonographic appearances of cystitis are summarized in **Box 2**.

ENDOMETRIOSIS

The urinary tract is not commonly involved in endometriosis; however, in women with a history of endometriosis, bladder involvement has been reported to vary from 1% to 15%.[12] The postulations for bladder endometriosis are (1) retrograde menstruation that seeds the surface of the bladder mucosa; (2) after surgery, especially after cesarean section; (3) metaplasia of mullerian remnants or direct extension from anterior uterine adenomyosis.[13] Bladder endometriosis can occur in several locations. Superficial and deep infiltrating lesions are more common in dependent sites in the peritoneal cavity. Imaging features can be nonspecific. However, the location of the lesions is more helpful in deciding in

the appropriate clinical setting. These masses may be inseparable from the uterus and may have variable protrusion in the bladder lumen. Transvaginal ultrasonography has been reported to be useful in showing the depth of endometriotic lesions in the bladder wall. MR imaging is superior to other imaging modalities because of its higher contrast resolution, delineation of bladder wall layers, tissue characterization, and multiplanar capability. These lesions may have a high signal on T2-weighted images, may show enhancement, and may also have a variable signal depending on the extent of fibrosis. Treatment of symptomatic bladder endometriosis consists of partial cystectomy.

URETEROCELE

A ureterocele is a submucosal cystic dilation of the intravesical portion of the ureter. The congenital defect is the obstruction of the meatus, and the ureterocele results as a sequela of hyperplastic response to the obstruction. Ureteroceles may be associated with either a single or duplex ureter. Ureteral duplication can be seen in approximately 75% of patients with ureteroceles.[14] Ureteroceles are most easily classified as intravesical, defined by their presence entirely within the bladder, or extravesical, which is seen as the permanent presence of the ureterocele at the bladder neck or urethra. Other classification systems for ureteroceles are based on the location of insertion of the ureter into the bladder, such as simple (insertion into the bladder) and ectopic (insertion outside the bladder).

A simple ureterocele can be seen on ultrasonography, a vesicouretherogram (VCUG), or an intravenous urogram (IVU). On ultrasonography, the ureterocele is seen as a cystic intravesical mass, contiguous with a dilated ureter and arising from a normally positioned ureteral orifice near the lateral margin of the trigone (**Fig. 7**). The wall of ureterocele is seen as a rounded structure located near the lateral margin of the trigone.[15] With real-time ultrasonography, partial or complete collapse of a simple ureterocele secondary to ureteric peristalsis can be shown. In these cases, further imaging should be performed to exclude a mass in the bladder. At VCUG, a collapsed simple ureterocele is usually seen as a rounded filling defect within the bladder. On IVU, a ureterocele is usually seen as a collection of contrast material within the ureterocele, thus producing a classic, cobra-head appearance consisting of a round or oval area of increased opacity surrounded by the radiolucent halo of the wall of the ureterocele.

Box 2
Sonographic appearances of cystitis

The wall is usually thickened and irregular. The wall thickening is usually most pronounced cranioventrally.

Thickening can be generalized or focal with trabeculated appearances and diverticulae formation.

In more chronic forms, bladder capacity is reduced.

In cases of tubercular and schistosomiasis, bladder wall calcification may be seen.

The urine may contain suspended or dependent echogenic material representing debris or calculi.

On sonography, it is difficult to differentiate various types of cystitis. However, in cases of emphysematous cystitis, intramural gas is seen as multiple hyperechoic foci with variable shadowing and reverberation.

In cases of hemorrhagic cystitis, blood clots are seen as mildly hyperechoic, nonshadowing, mobile material. The clots may settle on the dependent portion of the bladder.

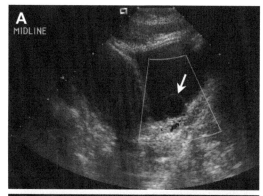

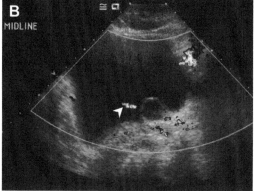

Fig. 7. Congenital ureterocele. Sagittal (*A*) and transverse (*B*) color Doppler images of the bladder show a cystic dilatation (*arrow*) of the distal end of the left ureter. Also seen is a left ureteric jet (*arrowhead*).

An ectopic ureterocele is a cystlike protrusion into the bladder lumen of the dilated, submucosal, distal portion of an ectopic ureter. It is usually associated with a duplex collecting system, and represents the distal portion of the ureter of the upper renal moiety. An ectopic ureterocele is more inferiorly located than a simple ureterocele. It is usually unilateral and seen much more commonly in girls than boys.[16] The sonographic appearance of an ectopic ureterocele is characteristic. The upper-pole collecting system of a duplex kidney is typically dilated and is connected with a dilated, tortuous ureter. At the level of the bladder, the hydroureter terminates in a round, thin-walled, anechoic intravesical cavity located out of the normal ureteral meatus. Further investigations, such as VCUG, should be performed for evaluation of vesicoureteric reflux into the proximal ureteral segments, and also for identification of bladder neck obstruction. In cases of complete duplication, an ureterocele associated with the upper-pole moiety is located medially and inferiorly to the lower-pole ureter, inserting in

a more superolateral location, also known as the Weigert-Meyer rule.

URINARY BLADDER HERNIA

Herniation of the bladder is seen in about 1% to 3% of inguinal hernias.[17] Most bladder hernias involve the inguinal and femoral canals, the femoral being more common in women, with a predilection for the right side. However, herniations can also occur through the ischiorectal, obturator, and abdominal wall openings. Any portion of the bladder may herniate, from a small portion or a bladder diverticulum to most of the bladder. The presence of a large bladder hernia with descent into the scrotum was termed scrotal cystocele by Levine[18] in 1951. In young infants, protrusion of the lateral aspect of the bladder base can be seen in the persistent, large inguinal ring, and is an incidental finding known as bladder ears.[17] The attributing causative factors of bladder hernia include urinary bladder outlet obstruction causing chronic bladder distension and contact of the bladder wall with the hernia orifices, loss of bladder tone with weakness of supporting structures, pericystitis and perivesical bladder fat protrusion, obesity, and the presence of a space-occupying pelvic mass.[19]

Bladder hernias are classified into 3 types depending on their relationships with the peritoneum: (1) paraperitoneal hernias, the most frequent type, in which the extraperitoneal portion of the hernia lies along the medial wall of the sac; (2) intraperitoneal hernias, in which the herniated bladder is completely covered by peritoneum; and (3) extraperitoneal hernias, in which the bladder herniates without any relation with the peritoneum.[20]

Most bladder hernias are asymptomatic and are discovered during surgery or during imaging procedures performed for other purposes. Bladder hernias can be seen on various imaging modalities such as excretory urography, retrograde cystography, CT, sonography, and MR. On excretory urography, a bladder hernia is seen as wide-mouthed, rounded protrusion of the bladder wall extending inferiorly. Bladder hernias may simulate a cystocele. However, these can be differentiated based on location of the protrusion on the bladder wall and on its direction. A cystocele is triangular and along the midline, whereas a bladder hernia protrudes laterally and inferiorly and is better depicted on oblique projection. Retrograde cystography is usually considered the best technique to image a bladder hernia. However, the hernia is visible only during voiding as a consequence of increased intravesical pressure. On CT, herniation can be diagnosed by identifying the position and the direction of the bladder. The most important sign is angulation of the base of the bladder anteriorly and inferiorly. Reconstruction along coronal and sagittal planes is also useful.[17] Sonography can also detect bladder hernias, although only inadvertently when large scrotal lesions are identified during routine ultrasonography for a scrotal abnormality. The bladder hernia is seen as a fluid-filled structure in the scrotum that can be followed cranially to join the intra-abdominal portion of the bladder (**Fig. 8**). It is not always possible to see the continuity based on the acoustic window. However, changes in volume of the lesion and thickening of its wall after micturition are the diagnostic markers.[21] MR imaging can be used for better depiction of the findings of other investigations. Sagittal and coronal planes show better relationship of the herniated bladder, especially in patients with large lesions.[22]

BLADDER FISTULA

The common causes of bladder fistulas are Crohn disease, diverticulitis, malignancy of adjacent pelvic organs, radiation or chemotherapy, iatrogenic causes, and trauma.

Crohn Disease

Crohn disease is the most common cause of ileovesical fistula and ileocolovesical fistula. Fistulas are slightly more common in men. The most common symptoms are pneumaturia, fecaluria, dysuria, pain, and fever.[23] The bladder is secondarily involved in adjacent bowel inflammatory lesions. Ultrasonography findings are usually nonspecific, and may show the presence of focal irregularity, wall thickening, or the presence of air within the bladder. CT is the most important imaging investigation. The common CT findings include air within the bladder, focal irregularity of the wall, and tethering of thickened adjacent bowel. The presence of orally administered contrast material in the bladder is the diagnostic imaging finding. Other imaging modalities to diagnose fistula include fluoroscopic studies of the bladder and bowel, such as small bowel series or cystography. Cystoscopy is the gold standard examination. Surgical resection is the treatment of choice.

Diverticulitis

Colovesical fistulas and cystitis are the known complications of diverticulitis. The common presenting symptoms include pneumaturia, pain, fever, pyuria, and fecaluria. CT is more sensitive

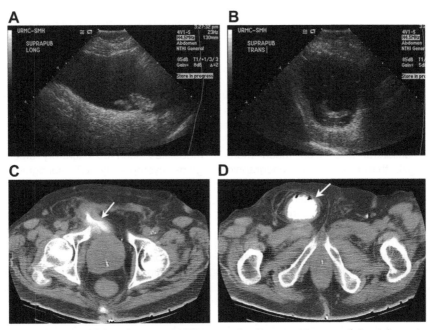

Fig. 8. Bladder hernia. Sagittal (*A*) and transverse (*B*) gray-scale ultrasound images of the right groin show a large cystic area with stones and debris within the right inguinal canal. Corresponding axial CT images from the delayed excretory phase (*C, D*) show a portion of the contrast-filled bladder (*arrow*) herniating into the right inguinal canal.

than cystography or contrast enema study.[24] The common imaging findings include bladder wall thickening with gas in the bladder lumen and adjacent inflamed colon with diverticula and pericolonic stranding. Left lateral wall of the bladder is the usual site of fistulas. The use of oral or rectal contrast agents opacifies the bladder and thus helps in establishing the diagnosis. Surgical excision of the fistulous tract and diseased bowel segment is the definitive treatment.

NEUROGENIC BLADDER

A neurogenic bladder is defined as urinary bladder dysfunction caused by neurologic trauma, disease, or injury. Risk factors for neurogenic bladder include various birth defects that adversely affect the spinal cord and function of the bladder, including spina bifida or sacral agenesis and other spinal cord abnormalities. Tumors within the spinal cord or pelvis may also disrupt normal nervous tissue function and place an individual at risk. Traumatic spinal cord injury is also a major risk factor for development of a neurogenic bladder.

Ultrasonography can measure the bladder volume. Normally, a bladder has a volume of 350 to 450 mL. Sonographic measurement of the postvoid residual urine is a commonly used noninvasive parameter for bladder outlet obstruction from any cause. At conventional or CT urography, or ultrasonography, the bladder is small and trabeculated, with an elongated appearance (**Fig. 9**). These findings reflect the major abnormalities in shape, size, and position of bladder, configuration of the urethra, the status of the external urethral sphincter, and competence of the ureteral orifices. The bladder neck may be dilated. Hydronephrosis may develop. On cystogram, the shape of urinary bladder in a neurogenic bladder has typically been called the pine tree, Christmas tree, or hourglass bladder.[25] This appearance is not pathognomonic of a neurogenic bladder and can be seen in patients with lesions anywhere along the sacral reflex arc, leading to poor detrusor compliance, or can also be caused by pelvic lipomatosis. In children, early adequate treatment can save the kidneys, and normal bladder growth can be achieved so that surgical bladder augmentation may not be required. Children with a neurogenic bladder are more prone to spontaneous rupture, catheter mishaps, and early rehospitalization for dehydration.[26] Bladder augmentation provides durable clinical and urodynamic improvement for patients with neurogenic bladder dysfunction refractory to conservative therapy.

BLADDER DIVERTICULA

Bladder diverticula are herniations of the bladder mucosa through bladder wall musculature

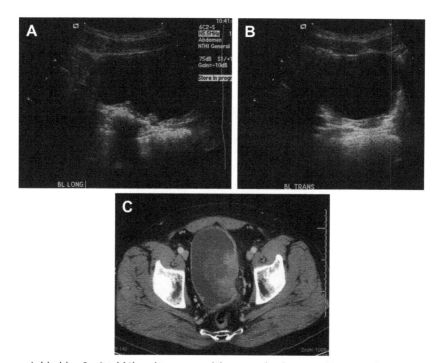

Fig. 9. Neurogenic bladder. Sagittal (*A*) and transverse (*B*) gray-scale ultrasound images of the bladder in a patient with spina bifida show an irregular and mildly thick-walled trabeculated bladder (*C*).

(detrusor muscle). Bladder diverticula most commonly occur lateral and superior to the ureteral orifices (**Fig. 10**). They may also occur at the dome of the bladder, particularly in such disorders as bladder outlet obstruction (ie, posterior urethral valves) or Eagle Barrett syndrome (prune belly syndrome). Depending on the size and location, bladder diverticula may cause ureteral obstruction, bladder outlet obstruction, or vesicoureteral reflux. Ureteral obstruction is unusual, occurring in approximately 5% of children with bladder diverticulum. Bladder outlet obstruction is rare. However, vesicoureteral reflux is more common, affecting 8% to 13% of patients.[27] Bladder diverticula can be congenital or acquired. Congenital bladder diverticula are usually associated with posterior urethral valves or neuropathic bladder. A diverticulum that occurs at the ureterovesical junction is usually called periureteral diverticulum, also known as Hutch diverticulum, and is often associated with vesicoureteric reflux.[28]

In male infants, bladder diverticulum must be differentiated from protrusions of the urinary bladder bilaterally into the inguinal rings anteriorly, known as bladder ears. These bladder ears are transient and usually disappear with age. Bladder ears are considered a normal variation, not a congenital anomaly. Bladder ears are lateral protrusions of the bladder through the internal inguinal ring and into the inguinal canal. In infants,

the bladder assumes a more abdominal position, which places it in close proximity to the internal inguinal ring. With growth, the pelvis becomes more developed, and the bladder assumes a more pelvic position. Therefore, this is rarely observed in adults. Bladder ears are often observed during VCUG or intravenous pyelography, when the bladder is filled to capacity. Bladder ears have also been seen on CT imaging. Lateral projections of the VCUG are essential to distinguish bladder ears from diverticula.

ACQUIRED DIVERTICULA

These are the result of obstruction, infections, or iatrogenic causes. They tend to be multiple and occur in trabeculated bladders (**Fig. 11**). Examples of causes of obstruction include posterior urethral valves, anterior urethral valves, urethral strictures, neuropathic bladder, and external sphincter dyssynergy.

VESICOURACHAL DIVERTICULUM

Vesicourachal diverticulum represents the caudal segment of urachus that fails to close, thus opening into the bladder. It can be congenital or acquired. The common presenting symptom is recurrent urinary tract infection. Sonographic appearances are fluid-filled structures extending from the bladder lumen, which may or may not

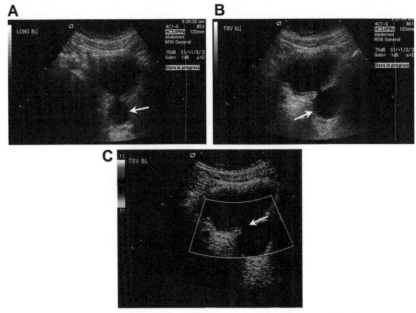

Fig. 10. Congenital bladder diverticulum. Sagittal (*A*) and transverse (*B*) gray-scale ultrasonographic images of the bladder show a large diverticulum (*arrow*) arising from the bladder. Corresponding color Doppler image (*C*) shows some color signal (*arrow*) at the neck of the diverticulum secondary to the flowing urine.

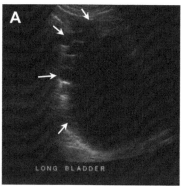
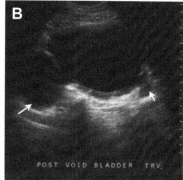

Fig. 11. Acquired bladder diverticula. Sagittal (A) and transverse (B) gray-scale ultrasonography images of the bladder in this patient with chronic bladder outlet obstruction show multiple bladder diverticula (arrows).

communicate with the bladder lumen. Vesicourachal diverticulum is an outpouching at the apex of the bladder that results from incomplete closure of the proximal urachus. Most patients are asymptomatic because the diverticula drain well with bladder emptying. Often, vesicourachal diverticula are incidentally discovered during evaluation for other reasons. Rarely, they become large and empty poorly, resulting in recurrent urinary tract infections or stone formation. Most bladder diverticula are diagnosed during evaluation for urinary tract infection, incontinence, or urine retention.[29] Diverticula are easy to diagnose on VCUG. With ultrasonography, these are seen as round to oval, anechoic fluid-filled collections that arise from the base of the bladder or around the ureteric orifice.

Complications such as stasis, infection, obstruction, and calculi formation can be seen. Development of carcinoma in bladder diverticulum is a rare, but known, complication.[29] There is a well-documented relationship between urinary bladder diverticula and bladder cancer. Intradiverticular tumors have a prevalence of 1% to 10%.[30] It is believed that urinary stasis produces chronic mucosal irritation and prolonged exposure to urinary carcinogens. Thus, there is a predisposition to malignant degeneration of the diverticular urothelium. The treatment of congenital bladder diverticula is surgical removal. Most acquired bladder diverticula, may resolve after relief of bladder outlet obstruction. Congenital diverticula are usually removed surgically.

FOREIGN BODIES IN THE URINARY BLADDER

There ware various types of intravesical foreign bodies. Usually, foreign bodies are self-introduced, the result of medical errors, have migrated from the surrounding organs, or are the result of a penetrating injury. Some are introduced by urologists, such as catheters (**Fig. 12**) and endoscopic instruments. Fragments of these

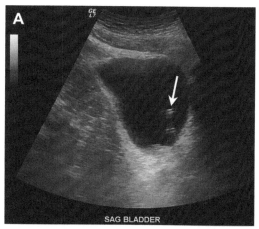
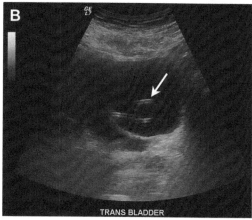

Fig. 12. Foley catheter within the bladder. Sagittal (A) and transverse (B) gray-scale ultrasound images of the bladder show the presence of Foley catheter balloon (arrow) within the bladder.

instruments, such as catheter tips, parts of catheter balloons, bougies, and the beaks of resectoscope sheaths, are some of the reported iatrogenic foreign bodies recovered from the bladder.[31] A variety of materials have been reported to migrate into the urinary bladder from surrounding pelvic organs, including an intrauterine contraceptive device, a vaginal pessary, an artificial urinary sphincter, and prosthetic slings. In some cases, these can be seen in patients with psychiatric illness. The other most common cause associated with intravesical insertion of bodies is sexual gratification. Complications of intravesical bodies include chronic and recurrent urinary tract, infections, acute urinary retention, calculus formation, obstructive uropathy, vesicovaginal fistula, and squamous cell carcinoma.[32]

Various imaging modalities can be used to identify and locate these foreign bodies. The most commonly performed initial radiological investigation is usually kidney-ureter-bladder radiography, which is helpful only in radiopaque foreign bodies. The use of abdominal and transvesical ultrasonography has been reported for the detection of nonradiopaque intravesical foreign bodies.[33] The degree of echogenicity of a foreign body is dependent on the disparity of acoustic impedence between the foreign body and surrounding tissues. Cystoscopy is the gold standard for confirming the presence, type, and location of the foreign body, and is also the most adequate method for treatment.[34]

INFLAMMATORY PSEUDOTUMORS

An inflammatory pseudotumor is a nonneoplastic proliferation of myofibroblastic spindle cells and inflammatory cells with myxoid components. Inflammatory pseudotumors have been described involving any organ of the body. Within the urinary bladder, the lesion is locally aggressive and may mimic malignancy either clinically, during cystoscopy, or during imaging. Inflammatory pseudotumors are not associated with smoking.[35] At imaging, an inflammatory pseudotumor usually appears as a single bladder mass, which may be exophytic or polypoid, and may also have ulceration. These masses usually spare the trigone, although large masses may invade through the bladder and may have a significant extravesical component, thus mimicking malignancy. On ultrasonography, these are seen as iso- to hypoechoic masses and they may show internal vascularity on color Doppler examination (**Fig. 13**). On CT and MR imaging, these pseudotumors show enhancement that is more marked at the periphery

because central portion usually has a necrotic component.

Treatment may consist of surgery, high-dose steroids, radiation therapy, or conservative management. It is important for the pathologist to differentiate inflammatory pseudotumor from malignant lesions, such as rhabdomyosarcoma and myxoid leiomyosarcoma, to avoid unnecessary radical surgery.

NEOPLASMS OF THE URINARY BLADDER

Bladder neoplasms can arise from any of the bladder layers. They are mainly classified as epithelial or nonepithelial (mesenchymal) tumors. Epithelial neoplasms are the predominant variety, with a reported incidence of 95%.[35] Epithelial tumors with differentiation toward normal urothelium are termed urothelial. The term urothelial carcinoma is used in preference to transitional carcinoma. Urothelial tumors depict a wide spectrum of neoplasia ranging from a benign papilloma through carcinoma in situ to invasive carcinoma. Other primary epithelial tumors include squamous carcinoma and adenocarcinoma, with rare varieties being small cell or neuroendocrine carcinoma, carcinoid, and melanoma. Because epithelial tumors arise from the most superficial layer of the bladder wall, they usually appear as irregular, intraluminal filling defects. Neoplasms arising from mesenchymal tissue differentiate toward muscle, nerve, cartilage, fat, fibrous tissue, and blood vessels. Benign tumors include leiomyoma, paraganglioma, fibroma, plasmacytoma, hemangioma, solitary fibrous tumor, neurofibroma, and lipoma. Malignant tumors include rhabdomyosarcoma, leiomyosarcoma, lymphoma, and osteosarcoma. Mesenchymal tumors originate from the submucosal portion of the bladder wall, hence often are seen as smooth intraluminal masses.

Urothelial Carcinoma

Urothelial cancer is the most common urinary tract cancer in the United States and Europe. Bladder cancer is more common in men than in women, with a ratio of 3 to 4:1. The most common presenting symptom is gross hematuria, although microscopic hematuria may be seen on urinalysis. There are various predisposing factors, including cigarette smoking, chemicals such as benzidine, naphthylamine, exposure to hair dyes, and drugs such as cyclophosphamide and phenacetin. Increased risk (2%–10%) of developing cancer has been reported in bladder diverticula.[35] Most urothelial tumors are located at the bladder base. They can be papillary, sessile, or nodular. Papillary lesions include papilloma, inverted papilloma, and

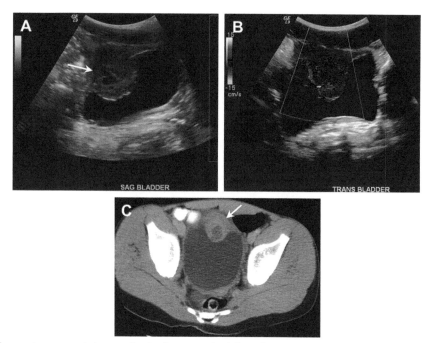

Fig. 13. Inflammatory pseudotumor. Sagittal gray-scale (*A*) and transverse color Doppler (*B*) images of the bladder show a heterogeneous mass (*arrow*) in the anterior wall of the bladder with presence of internal vascularity. Corresponding contrast-enhanced CT image (*C*) confirms the presence of an anterior bladder wall mass (*arrow*). Surgical resection confirmed it to be an inflammatory pseudotumor.

papillary urothelial neoplasms of low malignant potential. Sessile lesions include reactive urothelial hyperplasia, atypia, dysplasia, and carcinoma in situ.

Various imaging modalities are used for gross hematuria and suspected urothelial tumors. Ultrasonography can be used for the initial evaluation of hematuria. Most tumors appear as papillary, hypoechoic masses or focal wall thickening. Flow is usually seen on color Doppler imaging, which helps in differentiating these lesions from blood clots (**Fig. 14**). With CT or CT urography imaging, urothelial cancer appears as an intraluminal papillary or nodular enhancing mass or focal wall thickening. Tumoral calcification, although not common, can be seen in approximately 5% of cases.[36] The presence of ureteral obstruction is an indicator of muscle invasion. Increased attenuation or infiltrative changes in perivesical fat suggest extension of tumor into this site.

MR imaging has a superior staging accuracy of 72% to 96% for the primary tumor and also in detection of the superficial and deep muscle invasion compared with CT.[37] The usefulness of positron emission computed tomography in bladder cancer is limited because radioisotope is excreted into the urinary tract. However, it is helpful in detection of distant metastases and pelvic

recurrences, and also to differentiate tumor from postradiation fibrosis.[38]

Squamous Cell Carcinoma

Squamous cell carcinoma is seen in less than 5% of bladder neoplasm. However, the incidence is markedly higher in endemic areas affected with schistosomiasis.[35] Other risk factors include chronic irritation from indwelling catheters, bladder calculi, or chronic infection. The imaging findings are nonspecific. Tumors may be seen as a single enhancing bladder mass, or diffuse or focal wall thickening.

Adenocarcinoma

Adenocarcinoma is an uncommon bladder neoplasm constituting less than 2% of bladder neoplasm.[35] This neoplasm can be primary or secondary. Primary adenocarcinoma can be urachal or nonurachal, nonurachal being more common. Adenocarcinoma is associated with bladder extrophy and a persistent urachus. Other risk factors are intestinal metaplasia from chronic mucosal irritation, urinary diversions, and pelvic lipomatosis. Metastatic adenocarcinoma can be from contiguous involvement from colon, prostate,

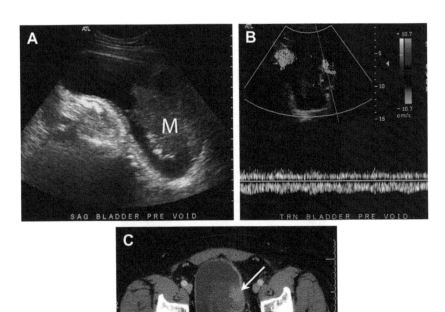

Fig. 14. Urothelial carcinoma. Sagittal gray-scale (*A*) and transverse color Doppler image with spectral analysis (*B*) of the bladder show a large mass (M) with increased internal vascularity. Corresponding contrast-enhanced CT image (*C*) of the bladder confirms the presence of a large mass (*arrow*), confirmed pathologically to be an urothelial carcinoma.

or rectum, and less commonly from lymphatic or hematogeneous route.[39]

Urachal carcinoma is typically located at the dome of the bladder in the midline or slightly off midline. These masses are seen as filling defects at the dome of the bladder or extrinsic compression. Sonographic features include heterogeneous soft tissue mass, which may show calcification and vascularity on a Doppler examination. CT imaging is the most sensitive method to show calcification and also extravesical spread, and is better than ultrasonography. Sagittal MR shows the location of tumor more accurately. On T2-weighted imaging, focal areas of high signal intensity from mucin are highly suggestive of urachal adenocarcinoma.[40]

Carcinoid

Primary carcinoid tumors of the bladder are extremely rare variants of neuroendocrine tumors. The most common clinical presentation is hematuria. Most are located at the bladder neck or

trigone region. Imaging features are not specific, the most common being intraluminal mass.[41]

Leiomyoma and Leiomyosarcoma

Leiomyoma is the most common mesenchymal tumor of the bladder, but constitutes only 0.43% of bladder tumors.[42] Bladder leiomyomas show characteristics similar to uterine leiomyomas, seen on ultrasonography as homogenously iso- to hypoechoic lesions. On MR imaging, the signal characteristics are intermediate on T1- and low signal on T2-weighted images. Increased T2 signal is usually seen in degenerated leiomyomas. Focal excision of the mass is the treatment of choice.

Leiomyosarcoma is the most common nonepithelial malignant bladder tumor in adults. An increased prevalence is seen after radiation therapy or systemic chemotherapy with cyclophosphamide for another neoplasm. It can be difficult to differentiate leiomyoma from leiomyosarcoma on imaging. However, large size, usually more than 7 cm, and more necrosis favor leiomyosarcoma. Treatment is radical cystectomy with resection of margins, combined with systemic chemotherapy.[43]

Rhabdomyosarcoma

Rhabdomyosarcoma arises from primitive muscle cells and can occur anywhere in the body except bone. Within the genitourinary tract, the bladder and prostate are the most common sites, constituting approximately 5% of all rhabdomyosarcoma.[5] Rhabdomyosarcoma is the most common bladder tumor in patients less than 10 years of age. It affects boys more than girls. Presenting symptoms include hematuria, dysuria, retention, and urinary tract infection. They are seen as large, nodular, polypoid filling defects or masses. On ultrasonography, they are seen as a homogeneous polypoidal mass. They are most often seen at the bladder base, and are sometimes difficult to differentiate from the prostate. With MR imaging, these masses show low signal intensity on T1-weighted images and high signal intensity on T2-weighted images. These tumors show heterogeneous enhancement. When they are multiple in the form of grapelike intraluminal masses, they are known as botryoid rhabdomyosarcoma.

Paraganglioma

Paragangliomas are uncommon bladder masses, constituting approximately 0.1% of all bladder masses. The age range is wide and there is a female preponderance.[35] In approximately 50% of cases, a characteristic clinical syndrome of severe headache, sweating, anxiety, pounding sensation, hypertension, and increased catecholamines can be seen during micturition, known as a micturition attack. Most of the paraganglioma are sporadic, but association can be seen in familial syndrome such as von Hippel-Lindau syndrome, Struge-Weber syndrome, tuberous sclerosis or multiple endocrine metaplasia, and neurofibromatosis. On imaging, these masses are usually solid, homogeneous, and well lobulated, but may have cystic areas caused by necrosis or hemorrhage. With ultrasonography, they are seen as an iso- to heterogeneous mass caused by necrosis. With CT and MR imaging they show marked enhancement. Typically, MR imaging shows low signal on T1- and moderately high signal on T2-weighted images.[44] Treatment consists of local excision following adrenergic blockade with lymphadenectomy if the lesion is invasive.

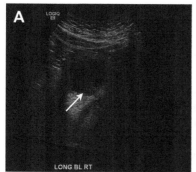
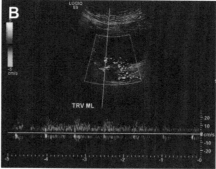
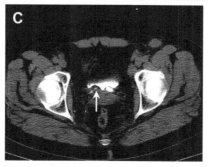

Fig. 15. Bladder lymphoma. Sagittal gray-scale (A) and transverse color and spectral Doppler (B) images of the bladder in a patient with known non-Hodgkin lymphoma show a small mass (arrow) at the right ureterovesicle junction. Corresponding contrast-enhanced CT (C) image of the bladder in the excretory phase confirms the presence of a small mass (arrow) at the right ureterovesical junction, with narrowing of the right distal ureter, presumed to be lymphoma.

Because there are no confirmed histologic criteria to distinguish benign from malignant tumor, long-term follow-up is required.

Lymphoma

Primary bladder lymphoma is rare because of the absence of lymphoid tissue in the bladder. Bladder involvement is usually secondary in patients with lymphoma and leukemia, and can be seen in 10% to 25% of patients (**Fig. 15**).[45] The most common occurrence for bladder lymphoma is in middle-aged women. The symptoms are nonspecific. The mass may occur at any location within the bladder, but most commonly at the dome or in the lateral walls. It is difficult to distinguish the mass from urothelial carcinoma.

Bladder Augmentation

Urinary diversion is a well-established urologic procedure. The indications of cystectomy are bladder cancer, end-stage bladder dysfunction such as from neurogenic causes, radiation damage, and interstitial cystitis. A urinary diversion is created by fashioning a segment of intestine into a conduit or reservoir to which the ureters are anastomosed. The 3 most common types of diversions are the incontinent conduit diversion (ileal or colonic), the continent cutaneous catheterizable reservoir (right colonic pouch), and the orthotopic neobladder.[46] Complications of urinary diversions include anastomotic leaks, hemorrhage, upper urinary tract infection, abscess formation, ischemia and obstruction, deterioration of renal function, and tumor recurrence.[47] Radiological evaluation of patients with urinary diversions to assess postoperative complications, particularly tumor recurrence, can be difficult and technically challenging. Excretory urography and fluoroscopic retrograde contrast injections of the diversion (fluoroscopic loopography or pouchography) historically have been the used in postoperative period. With the advent of CT, especially CT urography, this has become the most widely used modality.

Ultrasonography can be used to follow up the evaluation for hydronephrosis. Sonographic evaluation of the urinary tract after bladder augmentation and replacement procedures often reveals unexpected findings that result from incorporation of bowel into the urinary bladder wall. Familiarity with such findings is important to avoid misinterpreting them as abnormalities. The most common findings are thick or irregularly shaped bladder walls (**Fig. 16**), pseudomasses within the bladder lumen, and fine debris or linear strands. Pseudomasses are potentially the most confusing; they are usually attributable to normal bowel folds,

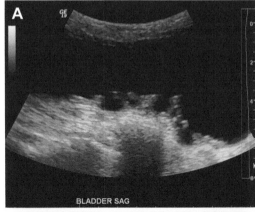

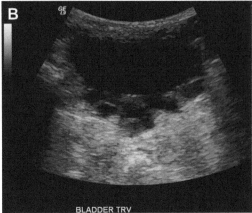

Fig. 16. Augmented bladder. Sagittal (*A*) and transverse (*B*) gray-scale images of the bladder in this patient after bladder augmentation for bladder cancer show an irregular wall of the bladder.

intraluminal mucus collections, or segments of bowel that have been intussuscepted into the bladder to prevent reflux.[48]

SUMMARY

Ultrasonography is an important initial imaging modality for the evaluation of the urinary bladder. Distension of the bladder is important for an optimal evaluation of the bladder. Several benign lesions of the bladder, including calculi, diverticula, and ureteroceles, can be detected with ultrasonography. Malignant masses of the bladder can also be diagnosed on ultrasonography based on the internal vascularity, thus differentiating them from blood clots. Some of the other lesions such as colovesical and vesicovaginal fistula are better and more accurately detected on CT or MR imaging. Staging of the bladder malignancy also requires additional imaging modalities. Ultrasonography may also have a role in the evaluation of the postoperative bladder.

REFERENCES

1. Klutke CG, Klutke JJ. Interstitial cystitis/painful bladder syndrome for the primary care physician. Can J Urol 2008;15(Suppl 1):44–52.

2. Verguts L, Deconinck K, Mortelmans LL. Alkaline encrusting cystitis. Urol Radiol 1987;9:53–5.

3. Wise GJ, Marella VK. Genitourinary manifestations of tuberculosis. Urol Clin North Am 2003;30:111–21.

4. Ghoneim MA. Bilharziasis of the genitourinary tract. BJU Int 2002;89(Suppl 1):22–30.

5. Wong-You-Cheong JJ, Woodward PJ, Manning MA, et al. From the archives of the AFIP: inflammatory and nonneoplastic bladder masses: radiologic-pathologic correlation. Radiographics 2006;26: 1847–68.

6. Crew JP, Jephcott CR, Reynard JM. Radiation-induced haemorrhagic cystitis. Eur Urol 2001;40:111–23.

7. Hanno P, Nordling J, van Ophoven A. What is new in bladder pain syndrome/interstitial cystitis? Curr Opin Urol 2008;18:353–8.

8. Ma JF, McClenathan JH. Emphysematous cystitis. J Am Coll Surg 2001;193:574.

9. Grignon DJ, Sakr W. Inflammatory and other conditions that can mimic carcinoma in the urinary bladder. Pathol Annu 1995;30(Pt 1):95–122.

10. Thrasher JB, Rajan RR, Perez LM, et al. Cystitis glandularis. Transition to adenocarcinoma of the urinary bladder. N C Med J 1994;55:562–4.

11. Capozza N, Collura G, Nappo S, et al. Cystitis glandularis in children. BJU Int 2005;95:411–3.

12. Batler RA, Kim SC, Nadler RB. Bladder endometriosis: pertinent clinical images. Urology 2001;57: 798–9.

13. Vercellini P, Frontino G, Pisacreta A, et al. The pathogenesis of bladder detrusor endometriosis. Am J Obstet Gynecol 2002;187:538–42.

14. Brock WA, Kaplan GW. Ectopic ureteroceles in children. J Urol 1978;119:800–3.

15. Zerin JM, Baker DR, Casale JA. Single-system ureteroceles in infants and children: imaging features. Pediatr Radiol 2000;30:139–46.

16. Berdon WE, Baker DH, Becker JA, et al. Ectopic ureterocele. Radiol Clin North Am 1968;6:205–14.

17. Curry N. Hernias of the urinary tract. In: Pollack HM, McClennan BL, editors. Clinical urography. 3rd edition. Philadelphia: Saunders; 2000. p. 2981–91.

18. Levine B. Scrotal cystocele. JAMA 1951;147: 1439–41.

19. Liebeskind AL, Elkin M, Goldman SH. Herniation of the bladder. Radiology 1973;106:257–62.

20. Reardon JV, Lowman RM. Massive herniation of the bladder: "the roentgen findings". J Urol 1967;97: 1019–20.

21. Catalano O. US evaluation of inguinoscrotal bladder hernias: report of three cases. Clin Imaging 1997; 21:126–8.

22. Bacigalupo LE, Bertolotto M, Barbiera F, et al. Imaging of urinary bladder hernias. AJR Am J Roentgenol 2005;184:546–51.

23. Solem CA, Loftus EV Jr, Tremaine WJ, et al. Fistulas to the urinary system in Crohn's disease: clinical features and outcomes. Am J Gastroenterol 2002; 97:2300–5.

24. Yu NC, Raman SS, Patel M, et al. Fistulas of the genitourinary tract: a radiologic review. Radiographics 2004;24:1331–52.

25. Ney C, Duff J. Cysto-urethrography: its role in diagnosis of neurogenic bladder. J Urol 1950;63:640–52.

26. Novak TE, Salmasi AH, Mathews RI, et al. Complications of complex lower urinary tract reconstruction in patients with neurogenic versus nonneurogenic bladder–is there a difference? J Urol 2008;180: 2629–34 [discussion: 34–5].

27. Blane CE, Zerin JM, Bloom DA. Bladder diverticula in children. Radiology 1994;190:695–7.

28. Pieretti RV, Pieretti-Vanmarcke RV. Congenital bladder diverticula in children. J Pediatr Surg 1999;34:468–73.

29. Zia-Ul-Miraj M. Congenital bladder diverticulum: a rare cause of bladder outlet obstruction in children. J Urol 1999;162:2112–3.

30. Golijanin DYO, Beck SD, Sogani P, et al. Carcinoma in a bladder diverticulum: presentation and treatment outcome. J Urol 2003;170:1761–4.

31. Habermacher G, Nadler RB. Intravesical holmium laser fragmentation and removal of detached resectoscope sheath tip. J Urol 2005;174:1296–7.

32. Schnall RI, Baer HM, Seidmon EJ. Endoscopy for removal of unusual foreign bodies in urethra and bladder. Urology 1989;34:33–5.

33. Barzilai M, Cohen I, Stein A. Sonographic detection of a foreign body in the urethra and urinary bladder. Urol Int 2000;64:178–80.

34. Granados EA, Riley G, Rios GJ, et al. Self introduction of urethrovesical foreign bodies. Eur Urol 1991; 19:259–61.

35. Murphy GD, Grignon DJ, Perlman EJ. Tumors of the kidney, bladder, and related urinary structures. AFIP atlas of tumor pathology, series IV. Washington, DC: American Registry of Pathology; 2004.

36. Moon WK, Kim SH, Cho JM, et al. Calcified bladder tumors. CT features. Acta Radiol 1992;33:440–3.

37. Tekes A, Kamel I, Imam K, et al. Dynamic MRI of bladder cancer: evaluation of staging accuracy. AJR Am J Roentgenol 2005;184:121–7.

38. Schoder H, Larson SM. Positron emission tomography for prostate, bladder, and renal cancer. Semin Nucl Med 2004;34:274–92.

39. Bates AW, Baithun SI. Secondary neoplasms of the bladder are histological mimics of nontransitional cell primary tumours: clinicopathological and histological features of 282 cases. Histopathology 2000; 36:32–40.

40. Rafal RB, Markisz JA. Urachal carcinoma: the role of magnetic resonance imaging. Urol Radiol 1991;12: 184–7.

41. Martignoni G, Eble JN. Carcinoid tumors of the urinary bladder. Immunohistochemical study of 2 cases and review of the literature. Arch Pathol Lab Med 2003;127:e22–4.

42. Binsaleh S, Corcos J, Elhilali MM, et al. Bladder leiomyoma: report of two cases and literature review. Can J Urol 2004;11:2411–3.

43. Rosser CJ, Slaton JW, Izawa JI, et al. Clinical presentation and outcome of high-grade urinary bladder leiomyosarcoma in adults. Urology 2003; 61:1151–5.

44. Crecelius SA, Bellah R. Pheochromocytoma of the bladder in an adolescent: sonographic and MR imaging findings. AJR Am J Roentgenol 1995;165: 101–3.

45. Bates AW, Norton AJ, Baithun SI. Malignant lymphoma of the urinary bladder: a clinicopathological study of 11 cases. J Clin Pathol 2000;53:458–61.

46. Stein JP, Skinner DG. Orthotopic urinary diversion. In: Reitick AB, Vaughan ED, Wein AJ, editors. Campbell's urology. 8th edition. Philadelphia (PA): Saunders; 2002. p. 3835–67.

47. Studer UE, Zingg EJ. Ileal orthotopic bladder substitutes. What we have learned from 12 years' experience with 200 patients. Urol Clin North Am 1997; 24:781–93.

48. Hertzberg BS, Bowie JD, King LR, et al. Augmentation and replacement cystoplasty: sonographic findings. Radiology 1987;165:853–6.

Ultrasonography of the Prostate: Update on Current Techniques

Ahmet T. Turgut, MD[a],*, Erkan Kismali, MD[b],
Vikram S. Dogra, MD[c]

KEYWORDS

- Prostate • Transrectal ultrasonography
- Benign prostatic hyperplasia • Prostate-specific antigen

Transrectal ultrasonography (TRUS) has tradition-ally been considered as the pivotal imaging test for the prostate, providing clinically important information regarding benign and malignant conditions, including benign prostatic hyperplasia (BPH), prostatitis, obstructive infertility, and pros-tate cancer (PC). Today, the main reasons for the referral of patients for TRUS are evaluation for PC and guidance for prostate biopsy.[1]

SONOGRAPHIC ANATOMY

In adulthood, the normal prostate has an average dimension of 4.0 to 4.5 cm, 2.5 to 3.0 cm, and 3.0 to 4.0 cm in transverse, anteroposterior, and craniocaudal axes, respectively.[2] It is wrapped by a thin pseudocapsule, which can hardly be distinguished from the surrounding fascial planes.[2] Anatomically, the neurovascular bundles perfo-rating the prostate capsule are critical because they are a major site of capsular weakness and potentially prone to tumor involvement. The TRUS appearance of the normal prostate depends on age. In young men, the hyperplasia of the glan-dular tissue is negligible, whereas in older men the prostate transforms into a larger gland with a more rounded shape because of the development of BPH.[2]

On average, 70% of the normal prostate is composed of glandular elements and the remaining 30% consists of fibromuscular stroma.[3] The glandular prostate is conventionally com-posed of an inner gland consisting of a transition zone and periurethral glandular tissue and an outer gland involving a peripheral zone and a central zone. TRUS usually enables the distinction of the transition zone, appearing anteriorly as a hypoe-choic zone, from the peripheral zone, which is echogenic and homogenous in echotexture compared with the rest of the gland.[2] The central zone, on the other hand, is hardly discernible from the peripheral zone in healthy adult men. The transition zone is a major site for hyperplastic changes, constitutes apparently a larger propor-tion of the prostate in older men, and can addition-ally harbor approximately 20% of PC. Notably, 1% to 5% of PC is located in the central zone.[2] The peripheral zone, being also the main site affected by chronic prostatitis, gives rise to approximately 70% of PC.[2] The transition zone cancers, on the other hand, can hardly be differentiated from BPH nodules by TRUS.

SCANNING TECHNIQUE

Today, biplane probes with a combination of end-viewing and side-viewing transducers enable mul-tiplanar imaging in semicoronal, axial, and sagittal projections during transrectal prostate scanning. Technically, transducers in 5 to 8 MHz range

[a] Department of Radiology, Ankara Training and Research Hospital, Ulucanlar Caddesi, Ankara 06590, Turkey
[b] Department of Radiology, University of Ege, School of Medicine, Universite Caddesi, Izmir 35100, Turkey
[c] Department of Imaging Sciences, University of Rochester School of Medicine, 601 Elmwood Avenue, Box 648, Rochester, NY 14642, USA
* Corresponding author.
E-mail address: ahmettuncayturgut@yahoo.com

Ultrasound Clin 5 (2010) 475–488
doi:10.1016/j.cult.2010.07.004

provide a clearer resolution for the gland periphery, which is critical for the accuracy of the sampling during the biopsy procedure. The air artifacts having a negative effect on the quality of the image can be avoided with the use of ultrasonography (US) gel over a latex condom applied to the probe. Self-administration of enema on the morning of the procedure helps in evacuating gas and feces, which is another factor that may cause distortion of the TRUS image. An accompanying digital rectal examination (DRE) can be helpful for revealing suspicious physical examination findings correlating with TRUS abnormalities. Most examiners prefer a left lateral decubitus patient position because it is well tolerated. Finally, a full urinary bladder providing a clear interface with the prostate base helps in better visualization of the gland. However, the authors' observation in clinical practice is that the bladder should not be overdistended because this may cause the occurrence of urinary incontinence during a concomitant biopsy procedure.

TRUS evaluation of the prostate is started with a systematic scanning in the transverse or semi-coronal plane, beginning from the level of the seminal vesicles adjacent to the prostate base and continuing down to the apical level with the demonstration of the glandular zones. Later, scanning in the sagittal plane is advocated not only to reveal any lobar asymmetry but also to confirm any suspicious finding detected on axial or coronal scanning. The prostatic and extraprostatic structures, which are evaluated in a systematic approach, are listed in **Box 1**. Importantly, the ellipsoid formula enables the calculation of the prostate volume by using diameters in orthogonal axes:

$$\text{Volume of prostate} = 0.52 \times \text{td} \times \text{apd} \times \text{ccd}$$

Box 1
Anatomic structures evaluated by TRUS

Outer gland

Inner gland

Anterior fibromuscular tissue

Capsule

Periprostatic fatty tissue

Periprostatic lymph nodes

Neurovascular bundles

Ejaculatory ducts

Seminal vesicles

Rectal wall

Urethra

---

where td, apd, and ccd represent the transverse, anteroposterior, and craniocaudal diameters of the prostate, respectively. In patients diagnosed with PC, estimation for prostate volume can be helpful when recommending an appropriate therapy.[3] The relevant estimation might also aid in the management of the patients who are not diagnosed with cancer because it may help direct patient therapy for obstructive lower urinary tract symptoms.[3] The transrectal approach for prostate US also enables the operator to perform various diagnostic and therapeutic interventions for PC thanks to the significantly higher resolution provided by the technique compared with the other routes of US scanning.[4]

PC

PC is the second leading cause of cancer-related death in men. Apart from being a major medical problem, it is also a significant public health issue that may cause significant economic burden.[2] Although early detection of the disease is crucial for proper management, insignificant cancers can also be detected in addition to the significant ones. Today, the major tools used for the diagnosis of the disease are DRE, serum levels of prostate-specific antigen (PSA), and TRUS-guided prostate biopsy.[5] At present, the positive predictive value of prostate biopsies based on DRE, PSA, and TRUS findings is low, and this results in a significant number of unnecessary biopsies. Hence, improvement of the accuracy of the diagnostic techniques for the diagnosis of PC is an apparent necessity.[6]

The most common indication for TRUS examination of the prostate is the evaluation for suspected PC. Apparently, early detection of PC is closely associated with a reduction in mortality, with the treatment of early localized disease being the only chance for cure. Before the widespread availability of diagnostic tools enabling early detection of the disease, such as DRE, TRUS, and PSA measurement, PC was frequently diagnosed at an advanced stage, causing the patient's death in a shorter time. Although a serum level of total PSA (tPSA) exceeding 4 ng/mL can imply the presence of PC, patients with BPH and inflammatory prostate disorders can also present with increased serum tPSA levels. The lack of specificity of serum tPSA measurement for PC screening has inevitably led to further efforts aiming to define an ideal protocol combining PSA, TRUS, and DRE to improve specificity without a reduction in sensitivity. Although TRUS is recognized as the cardinal method for biopsy guidance, its low positive predictive value in diagnosing malignancy has consistently been seen as a weakness.

Gray-Scale US

Since its first clinical introduction in the 1960s, a steady improvement in TRUS technology has been achieved.[7] Although there has been a consensus regarding the use of TRUS for the assessment of prostate size and biopsy guidance, its limited value in the early and accurate detection of PC and the determination of local tumoral extension still poses a great clinical challenge for its efficient use. Nevertheless, the gray-scale US technique enables outlining the zonal anatomy of the prostate, and the gland can be easily delineated by TRUS from the periprostatic tissues, including the rectum, neurovascular bundles, and fat.

Classically, a hypoechoic lesion in the peripheral zone can represent malignancy, although PC may less frequently have an isoechoic or hyperechoic appearance (**Figs. 1** and **2**A).[2] Today, the use of other less specific features is required for the diagnosis of PC because a significant proportion of contemporary PC is isoechoic. In this regard, asymmetry of either the echotexture or glandular margin may be helpful. Accordingly, a nonspecific echo irregularity or a bulge or irregularity in the outline of the capsule can imply the presence of PC.[8] However, about half the PC lesions are invisible under gray-scale US. Moreover, several entities like BPH, prostatitis, atrophy, hematoma, ductal ectasia, and prostatic intraepithelial neoplasia can mimic the gray-scale appearance of PC.[2,9–11] Another challenge for the evaluation of PC is that it is mostly multifocal; a solitary round

mass may also appear, although its appearance is less frequent. Morphologically, only 30% of PC may appear as a focal nodule (**Fig. 3**A), whereas the lesion is accompanied by an infiltrative component in about 50% of the patients (**Fig. 4**A, B) and an infiltrative pattern predominates in the remaining 20%.[10] A US pattern suggestive of advanced PC is a diffusely hypoechoic and heterogenous echotexture of the peripheral zone, which is either isoechoic or hyperechoic compared with the inner gland in a normal prostate (**Fig. 5**A). Small cancers usually have a hypoechoic appearance, whereas an enlargement of the tumor may result in transformation into an isoechoic lesion or one with an inhomogeneous echo pattern.[8] No specific US feature has been defined for transition zone cancers, although they are different from peripheral zone cancers in that they are less frequent and less aggressive clinically. Hence, systematic biopsy is the only means for the detection of transition zone cancers. The presence of a concurrent BPH may be a limiting factor during TRUS evaluation of the prostate because its mixed echo pattern or compression effect on the peripheral zone may mask PC.[12]

Apart from adenocarcinoma, the most commonly encountered histopathologic type of PC, the US features of the rarer prostatic tumors have also been described. Adenoid cystic carcinoma of the prostate can present with multiple uniform small cysts. Comedocarcinoma, being the most malignant form of PC, appears sonographically as a hypoechoic cancerous area interspersed with stippled multiple small hyperechoic foci. Lymphoma, on the other hand, has a US appearance of large hypoechoic masses in the transition zone and the peripheral zone. Finally, a soft-tissue mass infiltrating the bladder and prostate may be presenting a finding of rhabdomyosarcoma, which is a malignant tumor occurring during childhood.

Although the use of TRUS is limited for the staging of PC,[13] several TRUS findings may suggest an extracapsular extension. Among these findings are focal protuberance or irregularity of the prostatic capsule and hypoechoic stranding of the periprostatic fat planes. However, TRUS cannot reveal the extracapsular extension by small microscopic clusters of tumor cells.[14]

Color Doppler Ultrasonography

Doppler imaging is a means for assessing local blood flow, which is closely associated with tissue function and viability.[2,15] In color Doppler ultrasonography (CDUS), color assignment is related with the direction of blood flow and the orientation

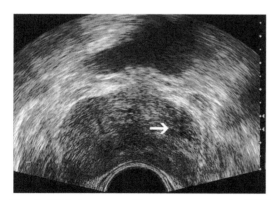

Fig. 1. Prostate cancer. Transverse gray-scale TRUS image showing ill-defined, slightly hypoechoic lesion with subcapsular location in the left lobe (*arrow*), which was histopathologically proved to be adenocarcinoma.

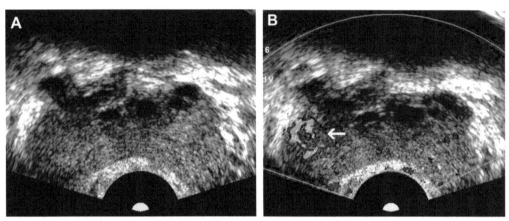

Fig. 2. Prostate cancer. (*A*) Transverse gray-scale TRUS image with no distinct lesion in the peripheral zone. (*B*) Transverse color Doppler TRUS image of the same patient showing an area of increased vascularization in the right peripheral zone (*arrow*), which was the only sign of histopathologically proved adenocarcinoma. The tumor was not apparent in gray-scale TRUS image because of its isoechoic nature. (*Courtesy of* Refik Killi, MD.)

of the transducer receiving the signal, where the flow toward the transducer is depicted in shades of red and flow away in shades of blue.[2] On the other hand, increased demand for blood in cancerous tissue with a growth rate faster than that of normal tissue may cause significant changes in local hemodynamics. Consequently, this has an effect on the visibility and detectability

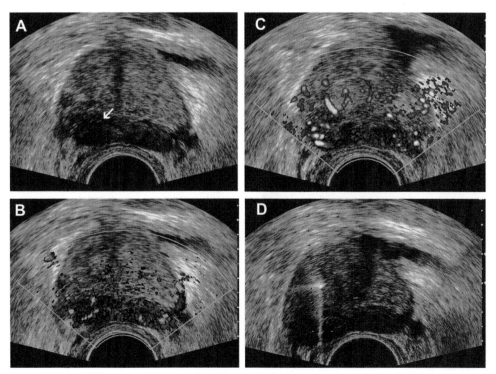

Fig. 3. Prostate cancer. (*A*) Transverse gray-scale TRUS image depicting a round, hypoechoic lesion located in the right peripheral zone (*arrow*). Neither color (*B*) nor power (*C*) Doppler TRUS examinations reveal markedly increased blood flow, which would represent neovascularity associated with PC. (*D*) Transverse TRUS image depicting the trajectory of the needle used for sampling the aforementioned lesion.

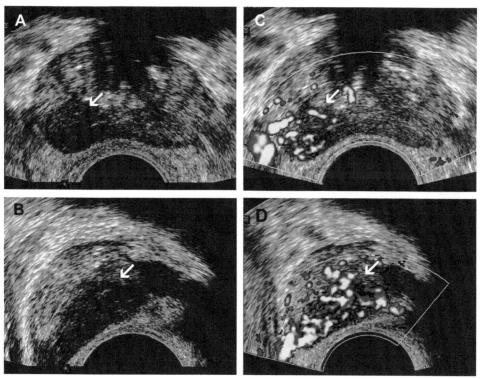

Fig. 4. Prostate cancer. (*A, B*) Transverse and longitudinal gray-scale TRUS images showing a focal nodule in the right peripheral zone (*arrows* in *A* and *B*). (*C, D*) Increased vascularization was detected in the lesion on transverse and longitudinal power Doppler TRUS images (*arrows* in *C* and *D*).

of cancerous sites by CDUS (see **Fig. 5B**).[16] In cancerous tissue, an increased number of enlarged and irregular blood vessels reflecting angiogenesis and an increased flow rate can be detected by CDUS (see **Fig. 2A**, B).[16] Technically, increased blood flow is shown either by spectral analysis in pulsed-wave Doppler imaging revealing waves representing the frequency shift or velocity or by color Doppler imaging depicting a spectrum of colors representing the range of mean frequency shift or velocities of red blood cells within the flowing blood.[17]

Earlier, it was believed that CDUS provided a better diagnosis of PC, where diffuse, focal, and surrounding patterns of flow can be encountered.[2] Later, it was realized that the specificity of the technique for relevant evaluation was low.[2] In addition, it was also noted that hypoechoic lesions implying PC and hypervascularity may not necessarily correlate (see **Fig. 3B**, C). However, it was shown that the color Doppler signal had a good correlation with the stage and the grade of PC and with the posttreatment risk of recurrence, which provided a clue for the behavior and aggressiveness of PC. Accordingly,

CDUS was helpful in the differentiation of low-risk, hypovascular tumors from high-risk, hypervascular tumors because the latter group was associated with hypervascularity representing a higher rate of Gleason tumor grades implying higher risk of extraprostatic spread (see **Fig. 5**).[18] Targeted biopsy solely depending on high-frequency color or power Doppler imaging is not recommended because of the theoretical risk of missing a significant number of cancers.[13] Apart from the quantitative assessment of blood flow, calculating microvessel density representing the distribution of microvasculature can be helpful for assessing the blood flow to the prostate by CDUS. Naturally, increased microvessel density being higher in metastatic tumors was found to be typical for PC.[19] Because core biopsy can underestimate the histologic grade represented by Gleason score, microvessel density can be used as an indicator of the prognosis of the disease.[20] Among the technical limitations of CDUS for the evaluation of the prostate are the angle dependency of Doppler flow, the intraprostatic noise mimicking increased blood flow, and its inadequacy in detecting low flow velocities.

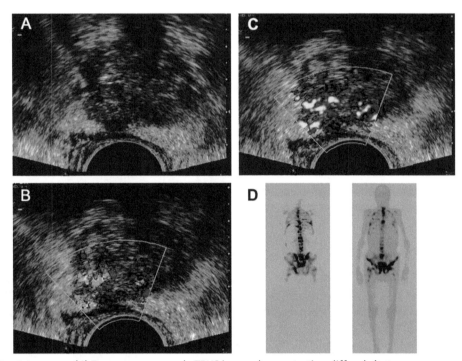

Fig. 5. Prostate cancer. (A) Transverse gray-scale TRUS image demonstrating diffusely heterogenous parenchymal echotexture with irregular capsular margin and marked posterior extracapsular extension; the lesion shows marked bulging and close proximity to the rectal wall implying infiltration by the cancerous tissue. Tranverse color (B) and power (C) Doppler TRUS images revealing increased vascularity of the lesion. (D) Whole-body scintigraphy of the same patient showing multiple areas of increased uptake in the axial skeleton representing pathologic osteoblastic activity, which is consistent with metastasis.

Power Doppler Ultrasonography

Power Doppler ultrasonography (PDUS) is less angle dependent than CDUS and provides color-coded information about the presence and intensity of the flow signals.[2] The technique has the advantage of detecting slow flow and even minor alterations in blood flow in small tumoral vessels (see **Figs. 4** and **5**).[2] However, the direction of the flow cannot be assessed by this technique. PDUS, which has a 3- to 4-fold sensitivity for the detection of PC, also aids in the differentiation of BPH and PC.[21] However, the technique was rarely reported to provide any benefit over CDUS for the detection of PC.[15] Although PDUS can help determine appropriate sites for prostate biopsy by identifying the areas of focal hypervascularity, the technique has not been considered to be superior to CDUS and was only reported to be useful for targeted biopsies when the number of biopsy passes was limited.[15] The combined guidance of gray-scale US and CDUS during TRUS-guided biopsy has not been found sensitive enough to preclude the need for systematic biopsy.[2] Recently, it has been reported that spectral

waveform measurements of the capsular and urethral arteries of the prostate by PDUS may be useful in differentiating PC from benign hypertrophy.[22] The investigators also speculated that an increased number of biopsy cores on the side with abnormal spectral Doppler index values would enhance the PC diagnosis.[22,23]

Contrast-Enhanced Ultrasonography

The microbubble contrast agents enabling the visualization of prostatic microvasculature can be helpful in better detection of PC because the increased microvessel density associated with angiogenesis in the cancerous prostate tissue is less than the resolution level of conventional Doppler imaging. However, most US contrast agents with a diameter less than 10 μm have the capability of penetrating even the smallest of microvessels. In this regard, contrast-enhanced ultrasonography (CEUS) enables the operator to image microbubble contrast agents. Thereby, the mismatch between the acoustic properties of the microbubbles and the surrounding blood results in intensified reflections of the ultrasound wave.[24]

Approximately 20 seconds after an intravenous injection, the number of US reflectors increases in the prostatic vasculature and this provides an improved Doppler shift signal yielding higher sensitivity for color and power Doppler measurements.[24] Maximum contrast enhancement occurs approximately 1 to 2 minutes after a single intravenous bolus, although the enhancement can be extended by intravenous infusion of the microbubbles. Time to peak enhancement, on the other hand, has been reported to predict the cancerous prostate lobe.[24]

In general, CEUS improves the sensitivity for PC detection without any decrease in specificity. CEUS may also provide a decrease in the number of cores to be sampled by enabling targeted biopsies. On the other hand, 3-dimensional contrast-enhanced PDUS with 3-dimensional image reconstructions before and after the administration of contrast agent and PSA levels has been claimed to be the optimal predictive combination for PC.[25] However, a major drawback for the clinical use of contrast-enhanced CDUS or PDUS is that the flow mainly in larger vessels is seen with the method because the microbubbles are destroyed by Doppler imaging before reaching the neovessels.[2]

Gray-scale harmonic US is another method for imaging the microbubble contrast agents. The method involves the use of lower energies for imaging contrast agents with less bubble destruction and greater penetration of the microbubble agents into microvasculature. Contrary to the contrast-enhanced CDUS technology, harmonic imaging techniques involve the detection of nonlinear responses of the bubbles. The phase inversion (pulse inversion) technology, using broad-bandwidth imaging, improves the assessment of the tissue perfusion by better detection of the signals reflected by the microbubbles.[24] Moreover, images with higher resolution are produced with the technique, contrary to the conventional US technology with narrow bandwidth, resulting in a loss of spatial resolution. Gray-scale harmonic US may increase the sensitivity for the detection of PC. Furthermore, higher degrees of enhancement have been shown to be associated with higher Gleason scores.[26] Intermittent imaging has recently been developed, which provides longer survival time of the microbubble contrast agents. Compared with the continuous harmonic imaging, intermittent harmonic technique provides a better parenchymal enhancement. Flash replenishment technique in contrast with harmonic imaging has of late been noted to improve targeting of sites with increased microvasculature during TRUS-guided prostate biopsy.

In a recent study conducted after premedication with dutasteride, a dual 5α-reductase inhibitor, before the prostate biopsy, a reduction of blood flow was demonstrated in benign prostatic tissues contrary to cancerous ones.[27] More recently, cadence-contrast pulse sequencing technology enhanced the observation of the microvasculature associated with PC, thereby improving the detection of PC.[7]

In general, CEUS improves visualization of PC thanks to the development of new microbubble-specific US techniques and better visualization of the microvasculature associated with PC,[28,29] although sensitivity and specificity are still not high enough to avoid systematic biopsies.[28] Although targeted biopsies together with systematic sampling protocols increase the detection rate, the role of CEUS in the routine clinical practice is questionable.[28]

Elastography

Elastography involves the evaluation of the elasticity of the tissues examined. Technically, the backscattered US signal changes little in degree if the insonified tissue is slightly compressed and decompressed during the examination. The compressibility of the insonified tissue has an effect on time or space differences between regions of interest with differing compression ratios. A specially designed TRUS probe is required for the application of the technique to prostate imaging. Technically, slight changes in the pressure applied to the prostate using the probe during TRUS examination result in changing the real-time image constructed, showing only the changes in local tissue compression.[8] Accordingly, a distinction can be made between cancerous and benign tissues depending on the hardness gradient and the degree of elasticity loss.[8] PC, characterized by limited elasticity or compressibility, is depicted sonographically as a dark zone. Hence, it has been considered to be a potential imaging modality for the detection of PC.[30] Although the use of elastography during TRUS examination can increase the detectability of PC by labeling the sites for biopsy cores,[3,30] it cannot preclude the requirement for systematic prostate biopsies, yet. The technique has also been noted to be potentially helpful in improving the staging accuracy of TRUS.[3]

TRUS-Guided Prostate Biopsy

The prostate biopsy procedure has been changed dramatically by the advances in TRUS technology. It has been agreed that TRUS-guided prostate biopsy is the gold standard tool for the detection of PC. The combined use of TRUS and needle biopsy has enabled directing the biopsy needle precisely into the target region and has resulted in an increase in the detectability of PC compared with digitally guided biopsy (see **Fig. 3**D).[31] Furthermore, prostate biopsy plays a pivotal role in the management of PC. The indications for TRUS-guided prostate biopsy are summarized in **Box 2**. Classically, abnormal DRE, elevated serum tPSA levels (>4 ng/mL), and suspicious finding on TRUS examination are the main indications for TRUS-guided prostate biopsy, although there is still no consensus on the upper limit for a normal PSA.[32] The procedure relies on a zone-based systematic sampling of the regions of the prostate, where the tumors are most likely to be located, because the disease has a multicentric nature and the diagnostic ability of TRUS alone for cancer detection is limited. Depending on the transducer design, sampling of the prostate is performed either in sagittal or axial scanning. Firing of the biopsy gun should be performed after indenting the prostate capsule with the biopsy needle so that contamination with the periprostatic tissue can be avoided and a longer tissue can be extracted during sampling.[32] In addition, the length of the needle trajectory within the gland should be predicted with the help of the trajectory line on an ultrasonographic screen so that inadvertent penetration of structures, such as urethra and periprostatic tissue, can be avoided.[32]

Because PC predominantly originates from the peripheral zone and that aggressiveness of the peripheral zone cancers is higher than those originating from the transition zone, the sampling approach should focus on the peripheral zone. The classical sextant biopsy protocol involves sampling of the cores midway between the lateral border and the median plane at the levels of the base, midgland, and apex of the prostate, respectively. Extended sampling protocols with 10 to 12 cores involving additional laterally directed cores at the aforementioned levels have been developed, although controversy still exists regarding the optimal sites and the number of biopsies. It has been reported that an increase in prostate volume has a negative effect on the diagnostic yield, with the number of cores remaining the same.[33,34] At present, the primary biopsies do not involve inner gland sampling because of their lower cancer detectability and lower metastatic potential of the inner gland. By means of TRUS-guided biopsy, Gleason grade, a measure of the aggressiveness of PC, can also be determined.

Preprocedural preparation and anesthesia
To minimize the risk of infection associated with the procedure, an antibiotic prophylaxis of Cipro (ciprofloxacin) beginning before the day of the procedure and continuing for 3 consecutive days is recommended.[32,35] In addition, the application of a bowel-cleansing rectal enema should be considered as a precaution against infectious complications, which would be helpful in obtaining a good TRUS image. A recent study has reported that patients with urethral catheter, with diabetes mellitus, or who are to undergo biopsy from more sites than 10 cores should be monitored after prostate biopsy because they would have had a greater risk of urinary tract infection.[36]

Because of an increasing concern for alleviating patient discomfort during TRUS-guided prostate biopsy, the application of several methods of anesthesia has recently become popular. Among these, periprostatic nerve block under TRUS guidance has been the most effective one and generally the most preferred.[37] After the penetration of the Denonvilliers fascia at the posterolateral aspect of the base of the prostate using a 22-gauge needle, the anesthetic agent (lidocaine without epinephrine) is infiltrated laterally at the white pyramidal site between the prostate and the seminal vesicle, which is also called the Mount Everest sign because of its white, peaked appearance created by the fat in this location on a sagittal plane.[32] Consequently, an ultrasonographic wheal is seen as hypoechoic filling of the Mount Everest area.[32] However, controversy still exists regarding the exact site, number, and dosage of the injections. More important, the injection of the anesthetic agent is preferably performed in the prebiopsy period to allow sufficient time for effect.[32] The technique might have some undesirable consequences, such as pain caused by puncture with the needle used for local anesthesia, the need for repeated

Box 2
Indications for TRUS-guided prostate biopsy

Abnormal DRE findings

Elevated levels of serum tPSA

PSA velocity greater than 0.75 ng/mL/y

Free PSA less than 20%, tPSA in gray zone

Ratio of pro-PSA to free PSA more than 1.8%

Suspicious TRUS findings

Before BPH surgery

To diagnose and stage recurrent prostate cancer after radiation therapy failure before salvage local therapy

injections during the biopsy procedure, systemic lidocaine toxicity, urinary incontinence, distortion or artifact formation on TRUS image, periprostatic infection, and erectile dysfunction.[38,39] In addition, the operator-dependent nature and the inefficiency of the technique in the presence of risk factors like patient anxiety, young age, repeat biopsies, or inflammatory anal diseases are among the disadvantages of the technique, where conscious sedation with intravenous midazolam would be an alternative and efficient means of anesthesia.[40]

TRUS in the Evaluation of Local Recurrence After Radical Prostatectomy

Radical retropubic prostatectomy (RRP) is an effective treatment for clinically localized PC. After RRP, recurrent PC is an important clinical problem in the long term in approximately 40% of patients, with more than 95% of the relapses occurring in the first 5 years.[41] Not surprisingly, the earlier detection of local recurrent cancer might allow patients to be treated with local radiotherapy at potentially more curable stages of the disease. It is well-known that the serum PSA should be less than 0.4 ng/mL within 2 to 3 weeks after RRP. In this regard, a rising PSA level implies local recurrence of PC at the prostatic fossa, metastatic disease, or a combination of both. In this regard, serum PSA has been the most useful tumor marker for monitoring patients with PC recurrence after RRP. Clinically, the diagnosis of locally recurrent PC is based on the combined use of DRE, TRUS, and TRUS-guided prostate biopsy.[42] In general, TRUS is considered to be a helpful procedure because it enables a precise evaluation of the normal and pathologic prostatic fossa anatomy. In patients with no clinical or biochemical evidence of local recurrence after RRP, TRUS typically depicts an appearance of a slitlike tapered profile extending from the bladder neck to the vesicourethral anastomosis (VUA), which is surrounded by a variable amount of hypoechoic tissue.[43,44] Specifically, a hypoechoic lesion next to the VUA, bladder neck, or retrotrigone is considered pathologic, although asymmetric thickening of the VUA or loss of integrity of the retroanastomotic fat plane should also be considered as suspicious for a local recurrence (**Fig.** 6A, B).[45] However, gray-scale TRUS cannot preclude the need for TRUS-guided prostatic fossa biopsy for a proper distinction between postoperative fibrosis and the recurrence of PC.[2] On the other hand, power Doppler TRUS, facilitating the identification of hypervascular areas within the tumoral tissue during TRUS-guided prostate biopsy, is considered to be helpful for the early detection of local recurrent tumors.[45]

BPH

BPH is a common disease among aging men, which involves the nodular hyperplasia of the fibrous, muscular, and glandular tissues within the periurethral glandular zone and the transition zone. The main role of US for the evaluation of patients with BPH is the assessment of the prostate size and postvoid residual volume (PVR) before the treatment. The technique can also be used for the assessment of the transition zone volume, which is closely associated with the

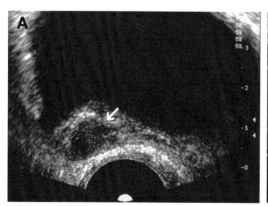
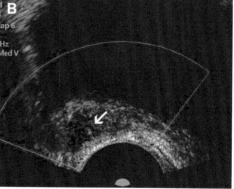

Fig. 6. Local recurrence after radical retropubic prostatectomy. (*A*) Transverse gray-scale TRUS image demonstrating an ill-defined, hypoechoic lesion in the prostatic fossa adjacent to the anastomotic region (*arrow*), which was later histopathologically proved to be recurrent adenocarcinoma. (*B*) Transverse color Doppler TRUS image of the lesion revealing areas of increased vascularization consistent with neovascularity associated with the tumor (*arrow*). (*Courtesy of* Refik Killi, MD.)

severity of BPH. Transabdominal US may have a role in the follow-up of patients with BPH because it is helpful in calculating the elevated PVR. Elevated PVR increases the risk for urinary retention. Furthermore, the upper urinary tract should also be investigated for any change.

The main TRUS findings in BPH are diffuse or nodular enlargement of the transition zone with hypoechoic or heterogenous appearance compared with the peripheral zone, bulging of the capsule of the prostate, cystic changes and calcifications in the adenomatous nodules, and compression of the peripheral zone by the enlarged transition zone.[46] Besides, associated changes in the proximal part of the urinary tract, such as elevation of the bladder base, increased PVR, bladder trabeculation, and hydroureteronephrosis, which are secondary to varying degrees of bladder outlet obstruction, can be detected. A surgical defect can be detected in the central part of the transition zone in patients with a prior transurethral prostate resection caused by BPH, which should not be misinterpreted as a cystic mass.[47] Cysts secondary to degeneration of the hyperplastic nodules associated with BPH are common in clinical practice.[47] Most importantly, protrusion of the enlarged transition zone should not be confused with tumors originating from the bladder base. An accurate differentiation can be performed by showing the discontinuity of the lesions and the prostate in sagittal TRUS scans.

PROSTATITIS

The term prostatitis is used for multiple prostate disorders causing pelvic pain, mostly having a nonbacterial etiology. Clinically, the entity has been classified as acute bacterial prostatitis, chronic bacterial prostatitis, chronic nonbacterial prostatitis, chronic pelvic pain syndrome, and asymptomatic prostatitis.[48] The role of TRUS is limited in patients with acute prostatitis because

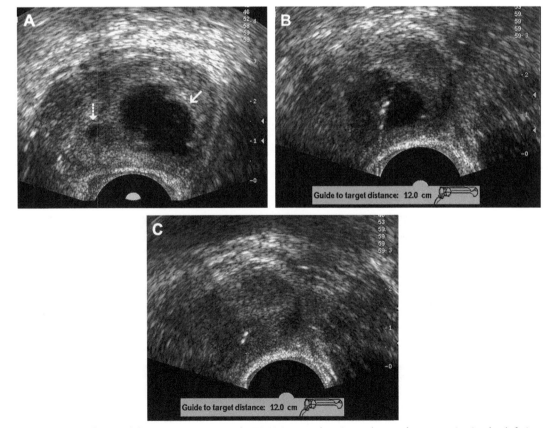

Fig. 7. Prostate abscess. (*A*) Transverse gray-scale TRUS image showing a large abscess cavity in the left inner gland with internal echoes (*arrow*), with an additional smaller collection in the right inner gland. (*B*) The external drainage of the lesion in the left inner gland was performed under TRUS guidance. (*C*) TRUS can also be used for the evaluation of the efficacy of the interventional treatment for the aforementioned abscess.

the diagnosis mainly relies on clinical evaluation. The patients having complaints associated with acute prostatitis, such as fever, pain, dysuria, urgency, and pyuria, even express significant discomfort during the insertion of the probe to the rectum because of severe pain and tenderness of the prostate. On TRUS, inflammatory findings such as a round, enlarged prostate with decreased echogenicity and diffuse hypervascularity on CDUS or PDUS can be seen. However, the main role of TRUS in acute prostatitis is to rule out abscess formation in patients who are unresponsive to treatment.[48]

Prostate abscess, occurring mostly in the fifth and sixth decades of life, is a rare complication of acute bacterial prostatitis.[48] The typical TRUS finding is a well-defined, thick-walled, uni- or multilocular fluid collection with internal echoes and septae, mostly located in the transition zone (**Fig. 7**A).[47,48] Apart from enabling the evaluation of the morphologic features of the abscess, TRUS also provides guidance for drainage of the lesion (see **Fig. 7**B). In this regard, drainage is recommended for an abscess larger than 1.5 cm, whereas antibiotic treatment is preferred for the smaller ones.[48] The follow-up involving the efficacy of either mode of treatment can also be performed by TRUS (see **Fig. 7**C).[48]

Chronic prostatitis, usually presenting with nonspecific lower urinary tract symptoms, appears sonographically as patchy, hypoechoic lesions or areas with heterogenous or increased echogenicity (**Fig. 8**A).[48] Increased vascularity of the aforementioned lesions on CDUS, dystrophic calcifications, capsular irregularity and thickening, dilated periprostatic veins, and periurethral zone irregularity can also be detected in patients suffering from this entity (see **Fig. 8**B).[47,48] Rarely, the prostate

can be involved in granulomatous disorders, resulting in an enlarged prostate with focal or multifocal hypoechoic lesions (**Fig. 9**A–C).[48] Tuberculosis is the most common type of infective granulomatous prostatitis, usually occurring secondary to the passage of the urine through the prostatic urethra. A concomitant involvement of the ejaculatory ducts may result in stricture formation. Because of the lack of specific TRUS findings, biopsy is the only means for a proper diagnosis.

PROSTATIC CYSTS

Utricle cysts and müllerian duct cysts are the most common midline prostatic cysts that can hardly be differentiated by clinical findings and imaging tools.[47] They may be silent or infrequently present with obstructive uropathy or infertility.[46] Müllerian duct cysts, which are usually larger than utricle cysts, are located slightly lateral to midline and may frequently have supraprostatic extension. Utricle cysts, commonly associated with abnormalities like hypospadias, cryptorchidism, or renal agenesis, can be diagnosed in younger men.[47] Rarely, PC can be detected in both types of cysts. A cystic cavity located at the midline and posterior to the urethra is the typical finding, although hypoechoic internal infectious debris can also be detected.

Less frequent ejaculatory duct cysts, occurring secondary to obstruction of the ejaculatory ducts either congenitally or secondary to inflammatory processes, appear sonographically as round or oval, thin-walled, unilocular cystic lesion with a paramedian location.[46–48] Rarely, they may cause a unilateral seminal vesicle dilatation.[48]

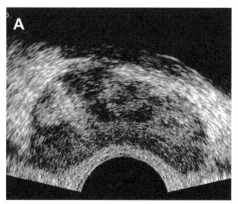 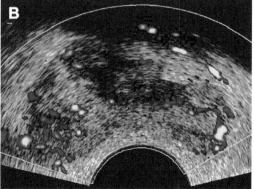

Fig. 8. Chronic prostatitis. (A) Transverse gray-scale TRUS image revealing heterogenous parenchymal echotexture with hypoechoic areas having patchy distribution. (B) Transverse power Doppler TRUS image of the same patient showing increased vascularization throughout the entire prostate. TRUS-guided systematic biopsy yielded chronic prostatitis histopathologically.

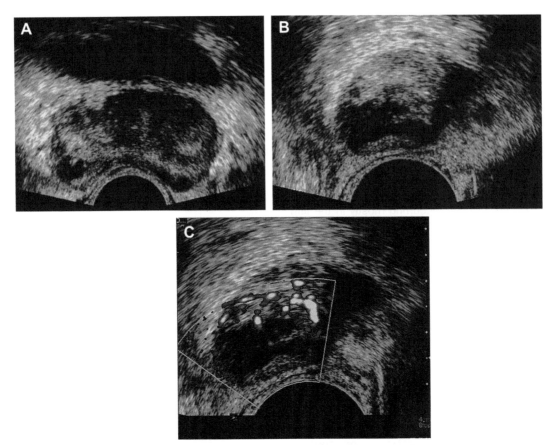

Fig. 9. Granulomatous prostatitis. (*A–C*) Transverse and longitudinal TRUS images showing an enlarged prostate with heterogenous parenchymal echotexture and multiple, randomly distributed, hypoechoic lesions. Colorflow Doppler reveals increased vascularity. TRUS-guided biopsy yielded granulomatous prostatitis histopathologically. (*Courtesy of* Refik Killi, MD.)

ACKNOWLEDGMENTS

The authors thank Professor Refik Killi, MD, for providing **Figs. 2, 6,** and **9.**

REFERENCES

1. Tamsel S, Killi R, Hekimgil M, et al. Transrectal ultrasound in detecting prostate cancer compared with serum total prostate-specific antigen levels. J Med Imaging Radiat Oncol 2008;52:24–8.
2. Turgut AT, Dogra VS. Prostate carcinoma: evaluation using transrectal sonography. In: Hayat MA, editor. Methods of cancer diagnosis, therapy and prognosis. 1st edition. New York: Elsevier; 2008. p. 499–520.
3. Boczko J, Messing E, Dogra V. Transrectal sonography in prostate evaluation. Radiol Clin North Am 2006;44:679–87.
4. Ukimura O, Gill IS, Desai MM, et al. Real-time transrectal ultrasonography during laparoscopic radical prostatectomy. J Urol 2004;172:112–8.
5. Heidenreigh A, Aus G, Bolla M, et al. EAU guidelines on prostate cancer. Eur Urol 2008;53:68–80.
6. Fuchsjager M, Shukla-Dave A, Akin O, et al. Prostate cancer imaging. Acta Radiol 2008;49:107–20.
7. Aigner F, Mitterberger M, Rehder P, et al. Status of transrectal ultrasound imaging of the prostate. J Endourol 2010;24:685–91.
8. Loch T. Urologic imaging for localized prostate cancer in 2007. World J Urol 2007;25:121–9.
9. Prando A, Billis A. Focal prostatic atrophy: mimicry of prostatic cancer on TRUS and 3D-MRSI studies. Abdom Imaging 2009;34:271–5.
10. Grossfeld GD, Coakley FV. Benign prostatic hyperplasia: clinical overview and value of diagnostic imaging. Radiol Clin North Am 2000;38:31–47.
11. Tamsel S, Killi R, Ertan Y, et al. A rare case of granulomatous prostatitis caused by mycobacterium tuberculosis. J Clin Ultrasound 2007;35:58–61.
12. Purohit RS, Shinohara K, Meng MV, et al. Imaging clinically localized prostate cancer. Urol Clin North Am 2003;30:279–93.

13. Carey BM. Imaging for prostate cancer. Clin Oncol (R Coll Radiol) 2005;17:553–9.
14. Papatheodorou A, Ellinas P, Tandeles S, et al. Transrectal ultrasonography and ultrasound-guided biopsies of the prostate gland: how, when, and where. Curr Probl Diagn Radiol 2005;34:76–83.
15. Halpern EJ, Sturp SE. Using gray scale and color and power Doppler sonography to detect prostatic cancer. Am J Roentgenol 2000;174:623–7.
16. Frauscher F, Klauser A, Halpern EJ. Advances in ultrasound for the detection of prostate cancer. Ultrasound Q 2002;18:135–42.
17. Jain SP, Fan PH, Philpot EF, et al. Influence of various instrument settings on the flow information derived from the power mode. Ultrasound Med Biol 1991;17:49–54.
18. Cornud F, Hamida K, Flam T, et al. Endorectal color doppler sonography and endorectal MR imaging features of nonpalpable prostate cancer: correlation with radical prostatectomy findings. Am J Roentgenol 2000;175:1161–8.
19. Hall MC, Troncoso P, Pollack A. Significance of tumor angiogenesis in clinically localized prostate carcinoma treated with external beam radiotherapy. Urology 1994;44:869–75.
20. Lissbrant IF, Stattin P, Damber JE, et al. Vascular density is a predictor of cancer-specific survival in prostatic carcinoma. Prostate 1997;33:38–45.
21. Cho JY, Kim SH, Lee SE. Diffuse prostatic lesions: role of color Doppler and power Doppler ultrasonography. J Ultrasound Med 1998;17:283–7.
22. Turgut AT, Olcucuoglu E, Kosar P, et al. Power Doppler ultrasonography of the feeding arteries of the prostate gland: a novel approach to the diagnosis of prostate cancer? J Ultrasound Med 2007;26:875–83.
23. Coley CM, Barry MJ, Fleming C, et al. Early detection of prostate cancer. Part I: prior probability and effectiveness of tests. The American College of Physicians. Ann Intern Med 1997;126:394–406.
24. Wijkstra H, Wink MH, de la Rosette JJ. Contrast specific imaging in the detection and localization of prostate cancer. World J Urol 2004;22:346–50.
25. Unal D, Sedelaar JP, Aarnink RG, et al. Three-dimensional contrast-enhanced power Doppler ultrasonography and conventional examination methods: the value of diagnostic predictors of PC. BJU Int 2000;86:58–64.
26. Halpern EJ, Rosenberg M, Gomella LG. Prostate cancer: contrast-enhanced ultrasound for detection. Radiology 2001;219:219–25.
27. Mitterberger M, Pinggera G, Horninger W, et al. Dutasteride prior to contrast-enhanced colour Doppler ultrasound prostate biopsy increases prostate cancer detection. Eur Urol 2008;53:112–7.
28. Wink M, Frauscher F, Cosgrove D, et al. Contrast-enhanced ultrasound and prostate cancer; a multicentre European research coordination project. Eur Urol 2008;54:982–92.
29. Aigner F, Pallwein L, Mitterberger M, et al. Contrast-enhanced ultrasonography using cadence-contrast pulse sequencing technology for targeted biopsy of the prostate. BJU Int 2009;103:458–63.
30. Pallwein L, Mitterberger M, Gradl J, et al. Value of contrast-enhanced ultrasound and elastography in imaging of prostate cancer. Curr Opin Urol 2007;17:39–47.
31. Soloway MS. Do unto others—why I would want anesthesia for my prostate biopsy. Urology 2003;62:973–5.
32. Turgut AT, Dogra VS. Transrectal prostate biopsies. In: Dogra V, Saad W, editors. Ultrasound guided procedures. 1st edition. New York: Thieme; 2009. p. 85–93.
33. Ozden E, Turgut AT, Talas H, et al. Effect of dimensions and volume of the prostate on cancer detection rate of 12 core prostate biopsy. Int Urol Nephrol 2007;39:525–9.
34. Eichler K, Hempel S, Wilby J, et al. Diagnostic value of systematic biopsy methods in the investigation of prostate cancer: a systematic review. J Urol 2006;175:1605–12.
35. Sadeghi-Nejad H, Simmons M, Dakwar G, et al. Controversies in transrectal ultrasonography and prostate biopsy. Ultrasound Q 2006;22:169–75.
36. Simsir A, Kismali E, Mammadov R, et al. Is it possible to predict sepsis, the most serious complication in prostate biopsy? Urol Int 2010;84:395–9.
37. Alavi AS, Soloway MS, Vaidya A, et al. Local anesthesia for ultrasound guided prostate biopsy: a prospective randomized trial comparing 2 methods. J Urol 2001;166:1343–5.
38. Turgut AT, Olcucuoglu E, Kosar P, et al. Complications and limitations related to periprostatic local anesthesia before TRUS-guided prostate biopsy. J Clin Ultrasound 2008;36:67–71.
39. Irani J, Fournier F, Bon D, et al. Patient tolerance of transrectal ultrasound-guided biopsy of the prostate. Br J Urol 1997;79:608–10.
40. Turgut AT, Ergun E, Kosar U, et al. Sedation as an alternative method to lessen patient discomfort due to transrectal ultrasonography-guided prostate biopsy. Eur J Radiol 2006;57:148–53.
41. Han M, Partin AW, Zahurak M, et al. Biochemical (prostate specific antigen) recurrence probability following radical prostatectomy for clinically localized prostate cancer. J Urol 2003;169:517–23.
42. Wasserman NF, Kapoor DA, Hildebrandt WC, et al. Transrectal ultrasound in evaluation of patients after radical prostatectomy. Part 1. Normal postoperative anatomy. Radiology 1992;185:361–6.

43. Goldenberg SL, Carter M, Dashefsky S, et al. Sonographic characteristics of the urethrovesical anastomosis in the early post-radical prostatectomy patient. J Urol 1992;147:1307–9.

44. Wasserman NF, Reddy PK. Use of transrectal ultrasound in follow-up of postradical prostatectomy. Urology 1993;41:52–6.

45. Tamsel S, Killi R, Apaydin E, et al. The potential value of power Doppler ultrasound imaging compared with grey-scale ultrasound findings in the diagnosis of local recurrence after radical prostatectomy. Clin Radiol 2006;61:325–30.

46. Torigian DA, Ramchandani P. Hematospermia: imaging findings. Abdom Imaging 2007;32:29–49.

47. Nghiem HT, Kellman GM, Sandberg SA, et al. Cystic lesions of the prostate. Radiographics 1990;10:635–50.

48. Langer JE, Cornud F. Inflammatory disorders of the prostate and the distal genital tract. Radiol Clin North Am 2006;44:665–77.

Ultrasound Contrast Agents in Genitourinary Imaging

Chris J. Harvey, MBBS, MRCP, FRCR[a],*,
Paul S. Sidhu, MBBS, MRCP, FRCR[b]

KEYWORDS

- Ultrasound contrast agents • Renal imaging • Kidney
- Microbubbles • Ultrasound

Ultrasonography (US) of the kidney accounts for a large proportion of the routine clinical work load because US is inexpensive, quick, safe, and easily accessible; US is often the preliminary investigation for many renal diseases. The development of ultrasound contrast agents (UCAs) has lagged behind that of computed tomography (CT) and magnetic resonance (MR) agents such that most investigators, on identification of a focal abnormality, refer the patient for a CT or MR examination. However, contrast-enhanced ultrasonography (CEUS) is a useful alternative. The role of CEUS in the detection and characterization of focal liver lesions is well established.[1,2] The renal applications of UCAs have increased and diversified since their introduction,[3–5] and recent guidelines have recognized their importance in the urogenital tract (**Box 1**).[1] UCAs are simple to use and are well tolerated by patients.[6] The imaging methods operate in real time, often allowing a diagnosis to be promptly made without exposure to ionizing radiation, the fear of claustrophobia, and at a lower cost than CT or MR imaging.

This article describes the renal applications and limitations of CEUS and its role in the imaging of the urinary tract. CEUS can be used to problem solve in renal pathology, providing a practical alternative that may frequently provide additional information not evident on other modalities.

UCAS AND IMAGING TECHNIQUES

UCAs consist of microbubbles of air or a complex gas (eg, perfluorocarbon gas) stabilized by a phospholipid or polymer shell.[7–9]

Microbubbles are similar in size to red blood cells, typically 1 to 10 μm in diameter, so they are small enough to cross capillary beds but are too large to enter the interstitial fluid. These properties enable the microbubbles to serve as pure intravascular agents, in contrast to CT and MR contrast agents, which are widely distributed throughout the interstitial space. Microbubbles are stable enough to survive passage through the cardiopulmonary circulation and allow sufficient time for imaging, typically 5 minutes after intravenous injection. The principal agent used in Europe is SonoVue (Bracco SpA, Milan, Italy). SonoVue is composed of a sulfur hexafluoride gas with a phospholipid shell. The microbubbles are metabolized by the liver (shell component) and the gas is exhaled via the lungs.

A typical contrast dose for an adult patient consists of 1 to 2.4 mL of a suspension of microbubbles in saline solution. Once prepared, the microbubble contrast agent is stable for several hours. This dose is manually injected into an arm vein, followed by a saline flush. They can also be administered as a constant infusion via a pump when a steady state blood concentration is necessary for quantitative studies. Contrast-enhanced

Declaration of interests: None.
[a] Department of Imaging, Hammersmith Hospital, Du Cane Road, London W12 0HS, UK
[b] Department of Radiology, King's College Hospital, Denmark Hill, London SE, UK
* Corresponding author.
E-mail address: chris.harvey@imperial.nhs.uk

Ultrasound Clin 5 (2010) 489–506
doi:10.1016/j.cult.2010.08.005

Box 1
European Federation of Societies for
Ultrasound in Medicine and Biology (EFSUMB)
recommended uses and indications of
ultrasound microbubbles in the urinary tract

1. Evaluation of anatomic variations mimicking a renal tumor (pseudotumor)
2. Characterization of complex cystic lesions and suspected cystic renal carcinoma
3. Characterization of thrombus within the renal vein and vena cava
4. Suspected vascular disorders, including renal infarction and cortical necrosis
5. Renal trauma and follow-up

   (1) Use in addition to Focused Assessment with Sonography in Trauma (FAST) and US

   (2) In low-energy trauma

   (3) Where contrast-enhanced computed tomography (CECT) is of poor quality because of artifacts

   (4) Follow-up of known injuries to avoid ionizing radiation of CT

6. Patients with contraindications for the use of CT and MR contrast agents
7. Vesicoureteric reflux:

   (1) Follow-up examination for reflux after conservative or surgical therapy

   (2) First reflux examination in a girl

   (3) Screening for reflux (eg, siblings, transplant kidney)

8. After radiofrequency ablation (RFA) or surgery of renal cell carcinoma (RCC)

   (1) Immediate assessment of residual tumor after RFA

   (2) Follow-up of previous ablative therapy to assess response and detect recurrence

   (3) To guide the ablation needle in lesions poorly visualized on unenhanced US

From Claudon M, Cosgrove D, Albrecht T, et al. Guidelines and good clinical practice recommendations for contrast enhanced ultrasound (CEUS) - update 2008. Ultraschall Med 2008;29:28–44.

US allows a quick, continuous, and repeated examination of the kidney for several minutes. There is no nephrotoxicity associated with a CEUS examination and UCAs are safe for use in renal failure and renal obstruction.

Microbubbles may be imaged on B mode, color, power, and spectral Doppler. Originally these agents were developed for rescuing Doppler studies that would otherwise have failed. However, the vast amplification of signal leads to artifacts such as blooming and saturation. These

artifacts can be minimized by reducing the sensitivity of the ultrasound system, reducing gain, and increasing wall filter and the pulse repetition frequency. With the improvement in ultrasound scanners, microbubbles are now rarely needed for Doppler rescue except in the assessment of renal artery stenosis and transcranial US.

Microbubbles have unique interactions with the insonating ultrasound wave. At very low acoustic power, microbubbles reflect the ultrasound wave. As the power is increased (mechanical index [MI]<0.2) they resonate at frequencies used in the diagnostic range (2–15 MHz) with production of harmonic signals. As the power is further increased (MI>0.7) disruption occurs. The use of low acoustic power allows real-time imaging of microbubbles with bubble-specific modes that are tuned to the harmonic signals produced by the resonating bubbles.

The low MI technique is almost exclusively used to generate an image because the technique minimizes microbubble destruction, allowing real-time observation for the duration of the presence of the microbubbles in the blood pool. Low MI pulse inversion imaging causes the normal tissue echoes to be suppressed, thus the baseline precontrast image appears dark. Most ultrasound manufacturers have a split screen display whereby a B mode image and microbubble-specific image can be simultaneously displayed. This split display is to allow the sonologist to interrogate a focal lesion or region of interest on the B mode image so that the lesion can be fully characterized throughout the whole contrast study. This technique avoids losing the lesion on the dark precontrast image when echoes from normal tissues are suppressed or when the lesion becomes isoechoic with the adjacent parenchyma during the CEUS. Echoes from the microbubble contrast material are enhanced and, as a result, all postcontrast administration echogenicity is caused by the presence of microbubbles. Lesions with high vascularity appear echogenic with respect to the adjacent renal parenchyma because this reflects the increased number of microbubbles in their vascular pool; nonvascular lesions appear black.

Quantitative methods can be applied to the kidney using low- or high-MI techniques.[10] Because microbubbles are pure blood pool agents, their transit through a region of interest can be followed using a low MI technique. A time intensity curve (TIC) (**Fig. 1**) can be generated and, from this, several indices can be derived, such as arrival time, time to peak intensity, area under the curve, and rate of washout. Alternatively, during a constant intravenous infusion of microbubbles, perfusion can be measured by applying a short high-MI pulse

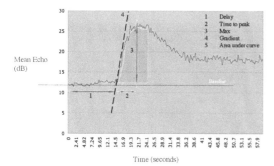

Fig. 1. Time intensity curve obtained from a region of interest (ROI) placed over the renal cortex following a bolus injection of microbubbles. A large number of quantitative indices can be derived from these curves. (*Courtesy of Dr Baxter, Glasgow Royal Infirmary, Scotland, UK.*)

to destroy the bubbles, followed by switching to a real-time low MI mode and recording the influx of bubbles. The resultant TIC (**Fig. 2**) exhibits an exponential increase in intensity obeying the equation $y = A(1-e^{-\beta t})$, where y is the intensity, β (gradient of the curve) is the speed of microbubbles, and A (plateau of the curve) reflects the blood volume/microvascular cross-sectional area. The product AB is a surrogate of perfusion.[11] Thus microbubbles allow a noninvasive assessment of the microcirculation and have been used to monitor blood flow responses to chemotherapy in RCC and derive prognostic survival indices.[12]

CONTRAST DYNAMICS IN THE KIDNEY

An understanding of the contrast dynamics within the kidney is essential to their use. In distinction

from iodinated and paramagnetic contrast agents, US microbubble contrast agents remain entirely intravascular and are not excreted by the kidneys, and therefore there is no nephrographic or excretory phase. The kidney has a single afferent blood supply and its enhancement pattern is different from that seen in the liver, which has a dual blood supply. Microbubbles do not stick to the vessel walls and therefore there is no late phase as in the liver. They are also not phagocytosed. The normal kidney takes 20% to 25% of the cardiac output, 90% of which supplies the renal cortex. Following an intravenous bolus of SonoVue, the cortical phase begins 10 to 15 seconds after injection and lasts 20 to 40 seconds followed by a slower medullary phase via the vasa recta lasting 45 to 120 seconds (**Fig. 3**). Initially, the renal pyramids are echo poor and slowly fill 30 to 40 seconds after injection and become isoechoic with the cortex in the medullary phase. The whole examination lasts about 2 to 3 minutes, which is shorter than the usual 5 minutes for a liver study. In addition, a lower dose of contrast agent is used (typically 1–1.5 mL) to avoid attenuation of the deeper parts of the kidney because of the high cortical perfusion.

CLINICAL APPLICATIONS
Renal Pseudotumors

Contrast-enhanced US is useful when evaluating normal anomalies of lobar anatomy that may simulate a tumor on baseline ultrasound. The column of Bertin[13] comprises nonreabsorbed

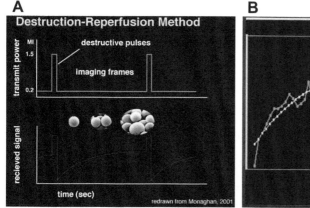
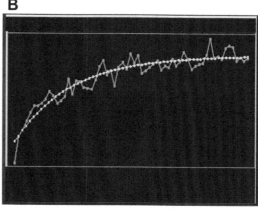

Fig. 2. Destruction-reperfusion technique. (*A*) Intermittent high-energy pulses of ultrasound are administered followed by a low acoustic power period during which the bubbles reperfuse into the region of interest. The lower trace shows how the intensity varies with time with a series of flashes (when all the bubbles are destroyed) followed by reperfusion curves. (*From Monaghan MJ: Contrast echocardiography. In Nihoyannopoulos and Kisslo, editors. Echocardiography. Springer; 2009.*) (*B*) The resultant exponential reperfusion curve is shown obeying the equation $y = A(1-e^{-\beta t})$, where y is the intensity, β (gradient of the curve) is the speed of microbubbles, and A (plateau of the curve) reflects the blood volume/microvascular cross-sectional area. The product $A\beta$ is a measure of perfusion.

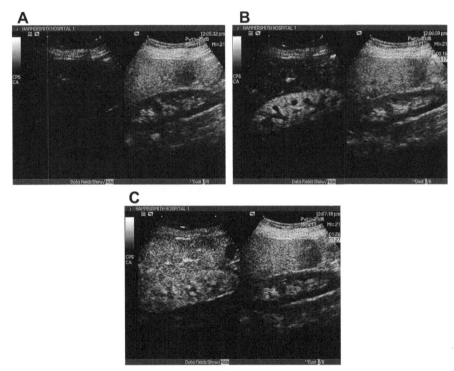

Fig. 3. Ultrasound contrast enhancement of a normal kidney imaged using low MI microbubble-specific mode cadence contrast pulse sequencing (CPS mode, Siemens, Mountain View, CA, USA). (*A*) On the precontrast image, the microbubble-specific image (*left side*) appears dark. The reference gray-scale image is seen on the right. (*B*) Seventeen seconds after SonoVue (Bracco SpA, Milan) injection, the cortex shows homogeneous enhancement with the pyramids and medulla seen as echo-poor defects. (*C*) One minute 27 seconds after injection. The pyramids and medulla have filled in and become isoechoic with the cortex.

polar parenchyma of 1 or both subkidneys that fuse to form a normal kidney. Its location between overlapping regions of 2 renal sinus systems, the presence of normal renal tissue, and the observation of a smooth surface contiguous with adjacent parenchyma is characteristic and reassuring. Fetal lobulation and lobar dysmorphism may also be misinterpreted as focal lesions.[14] In pseudotumors, the vascular branching is ordered, with no mass effect seen. Following administration of microbubble contrast, the suspicious area remains isoechoic to normal renal parenchyma in all phases of enhancement (**Figs. 4** and **5**).[15] Contrast agents can be given at the time the lesion is

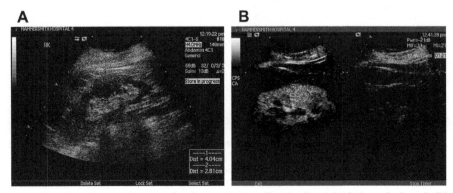

Fig. 4. Column of Bertin. (*A*) An echo-poor focal mass is identified in the right kidney (calipers). (*B*) Following administration of SonoVue microbubble contrast imaged using CPS mode (Siemens, Mountain View, CA, USA) this area enhances in an identical manner to the adjacent normal renal tissue, confirming benignity.

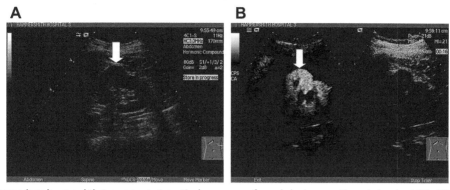

Fig. 5. Dromedary hump. (*A*) An apparent cortical mass was found during routine abdominal US. (*B*) Following administration of SonoVue imaged using CPS mode (Siemens, Mountain View, CA, USA) this lesion enhances homogeneously with adjacent normal renal tissue, consistent with a pseudotumor.

discovered, avoiding further investigation with CT and MR with beneficial cost and patient well-being implications.

Renal Cystic Disease

The Bosniak classification based on analysis of specific CT features is well established and has been adopted by radiologists and urologists in the assessment of renal cysts.[16] Simple (type I) or minimally complicated cysts (type II) are reliably assessed by B mode US appearing as a unilocular anechoic structure either within the parenchyma or renal cortex. Simple cysts remain dark following microbubble contrast enhancement even if they contain echoes on baseline ultrasound (**Fig. 6**). Hence, simple cysts, particularly small ones, are more conspicuous on CEUS, and this may be useful in the early detection of conditions such as polycystic kidney disease.

Renal cysts are commonly encountered lesions on US, CT, and MR imaging. Even on thin-slice CT

it can be difficult to identify the intracystic septations and nodules. Because of the superior spatial and temporal qualities of CEUS, real-time imaging of the microcirculation can be achieved, allowing resolution of flow within septa, nodules, and cyst walls that cannot be imaged on color/power Doppler, CECT, or CEMR. Hence, suspicious features such as septations or mural nodule enhancement that may not be evident on other modalities become more apparent (**Figs. 7** and **8**).[17,18] CEUS has been shown to be superior to unenhanced US and CECT in the diagnosis of malignancy in complex cystic renal masses.[19] In our practice, referral of incidental small or complex renal lesions seen on CT and MR for further characterization with CEUS is a frequent request. The Bosniak classification was originally based on CT findings but, because CEUS has been shown to be more sensitive than CECT,[19] some investigators have successfully adapted the classification and applied it to CEUS (**Table 1**).[17]

A practical use of renal CEUS is to evaluate those lesions that are equivocal for a benign/malignant

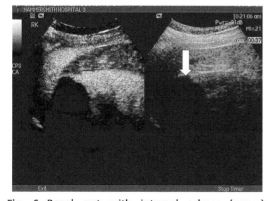

Fig. 6. Renal cyst with internal echoes (*arrow*). Following administration of SonoVue imaged using CPS mode (Siemens, Mountain View, CA, USA) the cyst showed no suspicious features with no internal flow. Appearances are consistent with intracystic debris or hemorrhage.

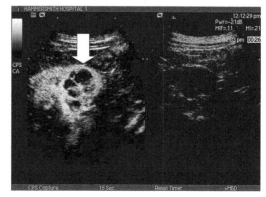

Fig. 7. Complex renal cyst. The B mode shows septation within a cyst. CEUS reveals enhancing thick septa and nodules (Bosniak type IV). A clear cell renal carcinoma was confirmed surgically (*arrow*).

A

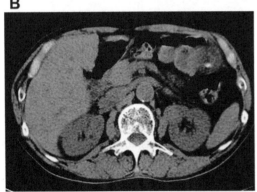

B

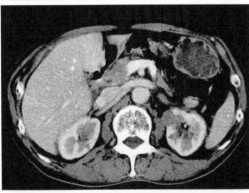

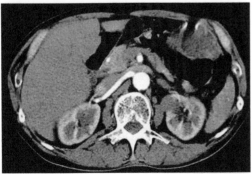

Fig. 8. Complex renal cyst. (*A*) CEUS reveals flow within a cyst (*arrow*) seen as internal echoes on the B mode image (*right side*). Compare this with the absence of intracystic flow in **Fig 6**. (*B*) CECT did not reveal any significant enhancing cystic lesions. A renal cell carcinoma was confirmed surgically. This case emphasizes the superior spatial resolution of CEUS compared with CECT.

Table 1	
Bosniak classification of complex renal cysts adapted to CEUS	
Type	**Features and Management**
I	Benign simple cyst. Thin walls with no septa, calcification, or solid components. No enhancement after microbubbles. No follow-up required
II	Few thin, hairlike septa with a few microbubbles seen in them. Fine calcification may be present in the wall or septa. Uniform high attenuation lesions (<3 cm in diameter) that are well defined and do not enhance after contrast. No further work necessary
IIF	Multiple hairlike septa that show a few microbubbles traveling along them. Minimal thickening of wall or septa, which may contain some calcification but no enhancement after contrast. No enhancing soft tissue components. Nonenhancing intrarenal lesions (>3 cm in diameter). These cysts are probably benign but need follow-up to show lack of change
III	Cysts with thickened irregular walls or septa that show enhancement on CT and CEUS. These cysts need surgical intervention. This group includes hemorrhagic or infected cysts and cystic neoplasms
IV	Frankly malignant cystic masses that have distinct enhancing masses separate from the wall or septa in addition to the features in type III. These masses require surgical resection

Adapted from Ascenti G, Mazziotti S, Zimbaro G et al. Complex cystic renal masses: characterization with contrast-enhanced US. Radiology 2007;243:160.

lesion on CT and MR (Bosniak type IIF, III, and IV cysts). This evaluation has become one of the most important applications of UCAs.

In overtly malignant cysts (Bosniak type IV), the main advantage of CEUS is in further evaluating the CT/MR findings. Microbubbles can be used to further characterize the tumor and distinguish solid from cystic and necrotic nonenhancing components.

RCC

The detection of RCC by ultrasound depends on its size, echogenicity, and whether it distorts the cortical contour. The sensitivity of US is poor compared with CT. However, US is responsible for the marked increase in detection of asymptomatic RCCs, which are in the region of 80%, and 30% of these are less than 3 cm in size.[20] The most difficult RCCs to detect on US are the isoechoic lesions, which do not exhibit mass effect or cortical abnormality. Color and power Doppler do not significantly affect the detection of small RCCs. CEUS can improve the detection of RCCs (**Fig. 9**), especially the isoechoic lesions, which may be more hypervascular than the adjacent parenchyma. The hypovascular RCCs appear as relative defects compared with the adjacent parenchyma (**Fig. 10**).[3] However, because microbubble agents only show the corticomedullary phase, and because tumors such as RCCs may present similar arterial phase contrast enhancement to the adjacent renal parenchyma, renal tumors may become less evident after microbubble injection. However, renal hypovascular metastases present a persistent hypoechoic appearance following microbubble injection, which may aid diagnosis.[21] Overall, CEUS is less sensitive than CT and MR imaging. Large RCCs require staging with CT or MR rather than CEUS, which may not add any extra information.

Currently, there are no exact enhancement criteria to distinguish between benign and malignant solid lesions, and varying contrast enhancement patterns may be shown in both benign and malignant tumors. As a result, the value of CEUS in renal tumor characterization is limited and presently CT and MR imaging continue to predominate. Although pseudotumors have homogeneous enhancement patterns identical to the adjacent renal parenchyma, true tumors usually show a disparity in enhancement. On CEUS, solid RCCs of less than 3 cm often show diffuse, heterogeneous, or, less commonly, homogeneous enhancement during the early corticomedullary phase, often with a hypervascular appearance.[21] Cystic or avascular necrotic components appear black, making them more conspicuous.

CEUS may be used to distinguish between those lesions that may be characterized on US alone,

such as minimally complicated cysts, hyperechoic or hemorrhagic cysts simulating a renal tumor, and pseudotumors, and those that need further cross-sectional imaging. As with cystic lesions, small (<3 cm) solid focal renal lesions are better characterized by CEUS than MR and CT because of the ability to show microflow within the lesions.

CEUS may increase diagnostic confidence for renal tumors in terms of lesion conspicuity and visualization of tumor vascularity.[4,22–25] Some studies have shown that diffuse enhancement of the lesion is a significant differentiating factor between benign and malignant lesions,[23,26] and other studies have shown that CEUS can improve visualization of the pseudocapsule of RCC.[27]

Xu and colleagues[25] retrospectively studied the CEUS patterns of 126 renal lesions (33 renal angiomyolipoma [AML] and 93 RCCs). On CEUS, the features of washout from hyperenhancement or isoenhancement to hypoenhancement in time, heterogeneous enhancement, and an enhanced perilesional rim achieved significant difference between RCCs and AMLs. Early washout and heterogeneous enhancement or peritumoral rim enhancement (which may represent a tumoral pseudocapsule) yielded the highest diagnostic capability in differentiating RCC from AML. The corresponding sensitivity, specificity, positive predictive value, negative predictive value, and accuracy were 88.2%, 97.0%, 98.8%, 74.4%, and 90.5% respectively. It was concluded that homogeneity of tumor enhancement and sustained enhancement are more characteristic of AML.

The current EFSUMB guidelines, published in 2008,[1] conclude that there are no specific patterns that reliably differentiate benign from malignant renal tumors on CEUS.

Because the sensitivity of CEUS is low in small renal tumors compared with CT and MR imaging, it should not be used in their detection. The exceptions to this are in patients with end-stage renal

A B

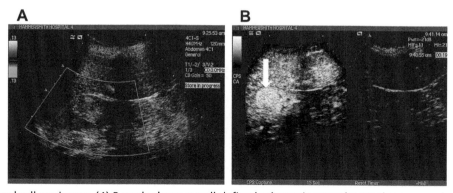

Fig. 9. Renal cell carcinoma. (*A*) B mode shows a well-defined echogenic avascular renal mass on color Doppler. (*B*) CEUS reveals avid arterial flow (*arrow*). An RCC was confirmed surgically.

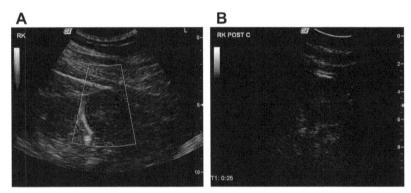

Fig. 10. Hypovascular renal cell carcinoma. (*A*) Color Doppler shows no vascularity in the renal mass. (*B*) CEUS shows minimal enhancement. (*Courtesy of* Dr Pilcher, St George's Hospital, UK.)

failure and Von Hippel Lindau[28] in which there is an increased risk of RCC.

CEUS and RFA

Percutaneous or laparoscopic RFA has become an accepted alternative therapy in RCC in patients who are unfit for surgery.[29,30]

RFA involves the image-guided insertion of a needle into the tumor mass followed by heating to achieve cell death. CEUS can be used in the context of ablative therapy and after surgery to (1) assess vascularity before ablative therapy in conjunction with CECT and CEMR, (2) immediately monitor the success of ablative therapies and detect residual viable tumor (**Fig. 11**), (3) follow-up of previous ablative therapy to assess response and detect recurrence, and (4) to guide the ablation needle in lesions poorly visualized on unenhanced US.

Renal Infarction

CEUS allows confident interpretation of renal perfusion defects down to the microcirculation.

On CEUS, perfusion defects appear as single or multiple focal wedge—shaped areas of absent, diminished, or delayed contrast enhancement compared with the adjacent renal parenchyma.[31] The defect is present on all phases of enhancement. CEUS is more sensitive than color/power Doppler in the depiction of infarcts, which consequently appear smaller on CEUS because the flow in the microcirculation cannot be shown on conventional Doppler modes (**Fig. 12**). Because of the increased sensitivity, CEUS can show infarcts when the kidney is deep or hypoperfused. CEUS is not hindered by the perpendicular flow of vessels in the renal poles that can cause problems in assessment of flow on color Doppler. Cortical necrosis is rendered more conspicuous by CEUS (**Fig. 13**). CEUS can reliably distinguish ischemia secondary to acute rejection or acute tubular necrosis from true infarction.

Renal Artery Stenosis

US contrast agents may be used in assessment of renal artery stenosis where they are used to aid

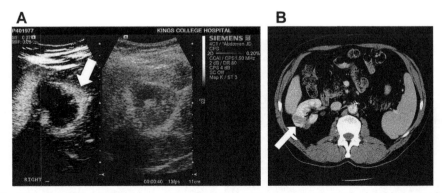

Fig. 11. After RFA of an RCC. (*A*) CEUS shows rim enhancement consistent with residual viable tumor (*arrow*) with central necrosis. (*B*) CECT confirms the presence of viable tumor (*arrow*). CEUS has the advantage that it can be performed immediately after RFA so that further treatments can be given.

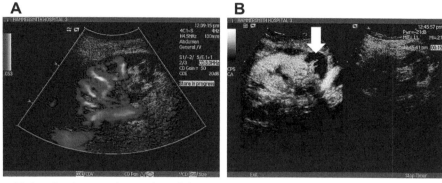

Fig. 12. Renal infarction in a renal transplant. (*A*) Power Doppler shows a large infarct. (*B*) CEUS reveals a much smaller infarct (*arrow*) because microbubbles allow the microcirculation to be imaged and therefore are more sensitive than conventional Doppler modes.

a Doppler study that would otherwise be nondiagnostic (**Fig. 14**). The sensitivity (71%–99%) and specificity (62%–99%) of Doppler US in the detection of renal artery stenosis has a large range in the literature because of the operator-dependent nature of US. It is a time-consuming technique with a high failure rate because the patients are commonly bariatric, there are multiple renal arteries in up to 25%, and the ostia of the main renal artery is not seen in up to 40 % of patients. US contrast agents improve the visualization of the main and accessory arteries, decrease the examination time, and increase the number of diagnostic studies.[5,32,33] Technological advances in modern US systems have resulted in marked improvement in the sensitivity of Doppler modes such that US contrast agents are not commonly used in everyday practice for the detection of renal artery stenosis. Instead, other functional applications are being used, such as measurement of the renal blood flow,[34] that may help in the patient selection for angioplasty and surgery. Time intensity curves can also be performed with measurement of peak enhancement and area under the curve, which are abnormal in the poststenotic kidney. These can be repeated after intervention to monitor the efficacy of the intervention. There is also potential for characterization of the plaque in the wall of the renal arteries, as has been successfully performed in carotid arteries.[35]

Renal Vein Thrombosis

CEUS can be useful in confirming or excluding renal vein thrombosis and distinguishing bland from tumor thrombus in RCC because tumor strongly enhances, whereas bland thrombus appears as a signal void in the vessel. CEUS can also help in assessing whether there is thrombus extension into the inferior vena cava. CEUS is also useful in assessing venous patency in renal transplants.

Acute Pyelonephritis and Abscess Formation

Acute pyelonephritis (APN) may manifest as a diffuse or focal inflammation of the renal parenchyma. US is often the initial imaging modality used in a patient with a urinary tract infection and suspected pyelonephritis. Diffuse pyelonephritis causes the kidney to enlarge and become echo poor with loss of corticomedullary differentiation. Focal pyelonephritis (sometimes called focal nephronia) may be seen as a focal echo-poor or echogenic area and may produce a masslike lesion mimicking a tumor. B mode has sensitivities ranging from 11% to 57% in one study.[36] Studies in animals and humans have shown an increase in sensitivity using UCAs compared with B mode.[37,38]

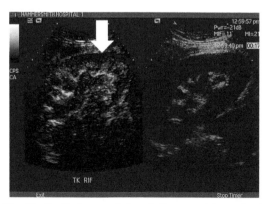

Fig. 13. Cortical necrosis in a failing renal transplant. CEUS reveals a thin rim of hypoperfused cortex (*arrow*) that was not seen on conventional Doppler mode.

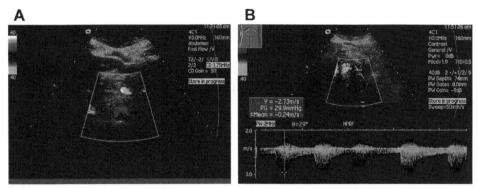

Fig. 14. Renal artery stenosis. (*A*) An axial section of the upper abdomen does not allow imaging of the renal arteries. (*B*) Following microbubble administration, the renal arteries were easily identified. Spectral Doppler interrogation shows spectral broadening and an increased peak systolic velocity (2.73 m/s) confirming renal artery stenosis. (*Reproduced from* Harvey CJ, Blomley MJ, Eckersley RJ, et al. Developments in ultrasound contrast media. Eur Radiol 2001;11:678; with permission.)

In another study, CEUS showed a sensitivity of 82% compared with 84% for CECT in the detection of pyelonephritis.[39] Although CT remains the gold standard for the diagnosis of APN, CEUS has a role to play as part of the initial US assessment in patients with renal obstruction or impairment in whom CT and MR contrast agents could have potential deleterious effects on renal function. CT imaging could be reserved for cases in which CEUS is negative and APN is still strongly suspected, or as a prelude to drainage.

APN is largely a parenchymal/interstitial process and the CT and MR signs of APN result from reduced interstitial opacification that is absent in CEUS because UCAs are pure intravascular agents. The defect of APN on CEUS may be subtle and not as clearly defined as on CT (**Fig. 15**). The conspicuity of the defect depends on the amount of edema and degree of focal vasoconstriction and vascular compression caused by the inflammation, and therefore there may be a spectrum between mild infection and abscess formation becoming more conspicuous on CEUS if APN progresses to an abscess.

There is usually complete absence of vessels and enhancement in the central liquid portion of an abscess as intralesion vessels are destroyed or displaced by the colliquative process. CEUS shows early rim enhancement followed by quicker washout compared with the adjacent normal renal cortex (**Fig. 16**). Internal septa are seen, which are more conspicuous on CEUS. The pararenal tissue may become hypervascularized.

Renal Trauma

In high-velocity trauma, CT is undoubtedly the modality of choice for assessment of visceral and skeletal injuries; however, in stable patients with low-energy blunt trauma, CEUS may have a role. Because there is no exposure to ionizing radiation, CEUS may be useful in renal trauma

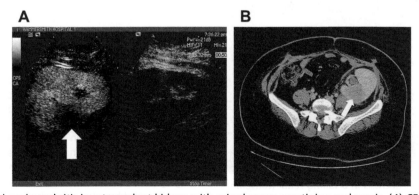

Fig. 15. Focal pyelonephritis in a transplant kidney with raised serum creatinine and sepsis. (*A*) CEUS reveals an area of relative hypoperfusion in the posterior cortex consistent with focal pyelonephritis (*arrow*). This cannot be seen on the B mode. (*B*) CECT confirms focal pyelonephritis (*arrow*).

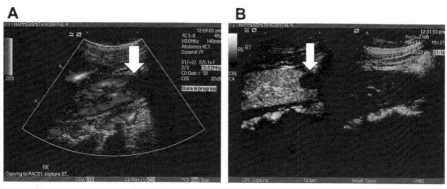

Fig. 16. 34 year-old woman presented with loin pain and pyrexia. (*A*) Power Doppler shows a defect in the lower pole (*arrow*). The differential is wide. (*B*) CEUS showed rim enhancement (not shown) and washout to form a spherical defect (*arrow*) consistent with a renal abscess. CEUS allowed the precise diagnosis to be reached.

(particularly in children), as an aid to the FAST scan in the emergency room, and for follow-up. A recent multicentre study in 156 patients found CEUS to be more sensitive than B mode US, and almost as sensitive as CT, in the detection of solid organ injury in blunt abdominal trauma.[40] Comparing B mode with CEUS, the sensitivity in the kidney increased from 36% to 69%. Valentino and colleagues[41] also found similar results in 133 trauma cases and concluded that CEUS was comparable with CT and also detected active bleeding. The kidney can be incorporated into a scanning protocol involving the liver and spleen. Generally, 1 mL of SonoVue is used and the kidneys scanned for up to 2 minutes, alternating between the sides, looking for bleeding, perirenal hematoma, and cortical lacerations. Normally, there is intense enhancement of the renal parenchyma following contrast administration. Hematomas or lacerations are avascular and appear as hypoechoic lesions on CEUS (**Fig. 17**). Current guidelines[1] recommend its use in isolated low-energy trauma, for which the CECT is of poor quality because of artifacts, and follow-up of injuries to avoid radiation exposure of repeated CT scans. CEUS allows a quick, continuous, and repeated examination of the solid organs for several minutes, can be performed at the bedside/emergency room/intensive care unit, avoiding ionizing radiation (especially in children), with no nephrotoxic problems, and at low cost.

Renal Transplant

In renal transplants CEUS can also facilitate the diagnosis of arterial and venous thrombosis and infarction with increased confidence and without any nephrotoxic effects. It is also useful in postinterventional complications such as bleeding, hematomas, arteriovenous shunts/fistulae, and pseudoaneurysms. In pseudoaneurysms and fistulae/shunts, CEUS aids in the demonstration of flow in deep-sited lesions and also in confirming complete thrombosis after treatment. CEUS is more sensitive than CECT or conventional angiography in the detection of perirenal bleeding and can show successful embolization and any adverse sequelae such as infarction. In recent years, there has been considerable research using microbubbles to measure renal flow in the post-transplant period, with promising results in monitoring graft function and directing antirejection therapy.[42–46]

Vesicoureteric Reflux

Vesicoureteric reflux (VUR) is the most common urinary tract abnormality in children, with an incidence of 1% to 2% in the general population[47,48] and a 30% to 50% incidence in children with recurrent urinary tract infections. Diagnostic imaging for VUR encompasses both radiologic and sonographic modalities. Radiologic modalities comprise voiding cystourethrography (VCUG), the most widespread method for examination for reflux, and radionuclide cystography (RNC). The sonographic diagnosis of VUR using intravesical administration of a US contrast agent (voiding urosonography [VUS]) is being increasingly used in the routine diagnostic imaging work-up and follow-up of reflux, because of the absence of radiation. VUS was first performed in the mid-1990s and is now the most common CEUS performed in children.[49] VUS was initially performed with Levovist (Schering AG, Germany) but studies have shown that SonoVue can also be used with good results, although it has not been licensed for clinical use.[48–51] It may be used on its own or along with VCUG and RNC in the investigation of reflux.

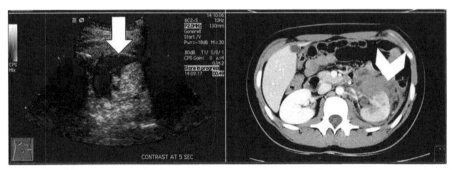

Fig. 17. Trauma. CEUS shows a perinephric hematoma around an irregular lacerated segment of devitalized kidney (*arrow*). CT confirms the CEUS findings (*chevron*).

The procedure can be performed via a transurethral catheter or suprapubic catheter/puncture.[1,52] A precontrast scan is initially performed. The contrast agent is then introduced into the bladder (Levovist concentration 300 mg/mL, 5% to 10% of bladder volume; SonoVue, less than 1% of bladder volume). Postcontrast scans are performed during contrast administration, paying particular attention to the terminal ureters and renal pelvis (**Fig. 18**). US is then performed during and after voiding. Urethrosonography can be performed in boys and girls with excellent results. The degree of reflux can be graded from 1 to 5, similarly to that used in VCUG. Scanning can be performed in fundamental mode, color Doppler, harmonic, or contrast-specific modes according to the contrast agent used. The procedure has been shown to be extremely safe, with no adverse effects reported. VUS has the potential of more than a 50% reduction in the number of children undergoing reflux examinations using ionizing radiation.[47]

Comparative studies show that VUS has a higher sensitivity than VCUG.[48,50,51] A meta-analysis[52] showed that, in 19% of pelviureteric units (PUUs), the diagnosis of reflux was made only by VUS, and in 10% only by VCUG. Thus, in 9% of PUUs, more refluxes were detected using VUS. In 73.6%, the reflux grades were concordant in VUS and VCUG. Reflux grade was found to be higher with VUS than with VCUG in 19.6% of PUUs. In 71.2% of PUUs with grade I reflux on VCUG, the reflux was found to be grade II and higher on VUS. Using VCUG as the reference, the results of VUS were as follows: sensitivity 57% to 100%, specificity 85% to 100%, positive/negative predictive values 58% to 100%/87% to 100%, respectively, and diagnostic accuracy 78% to 96%. With the exception of 2 studies, the diagnostic accuracy reported was 90% and greater. Comparative studies of VUS versus direct radionuclide cystography are too few to allow definite conclusions. The common selection criteria for VUS as the primary examination for VUR currently include (1) follow-up studies after conservative or surgical therapy, (2) first examination for VUR in girls, and (3) screening high-risk patients' (eg, siblings and transplant kidney). Limitations include the first reflux examination in boys because of the difficulty of excluding posterior urethral valves. Although scanning the urethra is

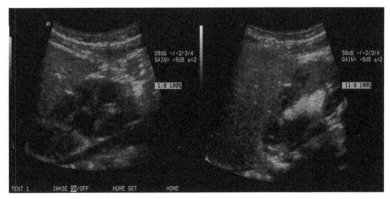

Fig. 18. VUR in a 3-year-old girl. Echogenic microbubbles are seen to reflux into a prominent renal pelvis during micturition on the right-hand image. (*Courtesy of* Dr Ruth Williamson, Hammersmith Hospital, UK.)

possible, it is not routinely performed. Bladder function cannot be assessed on VUS and VUS cannot be performed if the bladder and kidneys cannot be adequately seen on ultrasound (eg, in severe scoliosis).

Prostate Cancer

Transrectal ultrasonography (TRUS) remains the first modality of choice for imaging the prostate. However, gray-scale US has an accuracy of only 50% to 60% for the detection of prostate cancer and has an even lower accuracy for staging. TRUS is limited in detecting prostate cancer because of the variability in US appearances, the poor specificity of sonographic abnormalities, tumors frequently being multifocal, and the significant proportion of isoechoic cancers that cannot be differentiated from benign changes.

Angiogenesis is essential for tumor growth and invasion. Pathologic examinations of prostate tumors have confirmed the presence of angiogenesis within prostate carcinoma by showing increased microvessel density compared with the surrounding normal parenchyma.[53]

Imaging techniques that allow quantification of blood flow in these microvessels may provide the opportunity to significantly improve prostate cancer detection and characterization.[54] Despite changes in biopsy practice, and technological advances with the use of higher frequencies, broad band, and harmonic imaging, which have improved detection rates, there are still significant false-positive rates that have prompted the evaluation of Doppler imaging and microbubble contrast agents (**Fig. 19**) to ascertain whether targeted biopsies could replace systematic biopsies in the hope of reducing potential adverse effects of multicore systematic biopsy schemes.

Tumor vessels are of the order of 10 to 50 μm in diameter, which is considerably less than the 1-mm resolution limit of conventional Doppler techniques. Microbubble-specific techniques allow imaging of vessels as small as 50 to 100 μm in diameter.[55,56] In addition, because microbubbles are vascular tracers, following a bolus injection, their passage through a tissue of interest can be quantified to generate TICs from which many functional indices[10,56–58] can be derived, including bolus arrival time, time to peak intensity, area under the curve, wash in/out curves, as well as more complex deconvolution indices. The indices derived can be used to construct true functional images by displaying them on a pixel-by-pixel basis as an overlay on the gray-scale image (**Fig. 20**).[57] Grossen and

colleagues[58] showed that the time to peak enhancement was the most predictive parameter for the localization of the malignant lobe of the prostate, with 78% of patients correctly diagnosed. Quantitative methods can be used based on the destruction of microbubbles and observing the effects on contrast enhancement (reperfusion kinetics). Intermittent high-power ultrasound pulses may be used to destroy microbubbles within a beam, and the rate of replenishment in the field can be used to calculate microbubble flow rate, a surrogate of perfusion and fractional vascular volume.[11]

Rickards and colleagues[59] showed that the use of microbubbles increased the sensitivity, but decreased the specificity, in a series of sextant biopsies in 22 patients. Halpern and colleagues,[60] using contrast-enhanced real-time and intermittent harmonic imaging in addition to power Doppler, showed a significant increase in sensitivity from 38% to 65%, whereas specificity was maintained at 80%. These results have been supported by other workers.[61] Using a Levovist contrast agent and color Doppler–based targeted biopsy protocol, Frauscher and colleagues[62] showed that positive biopsy rates were significantly improved with targeted cores versus sextant cores (13% vs 4.9%, respectively). In a study of 230 patients, comparing contrast-enhanced biopsies with sextant biopsies, targeted biopsies were again found to be superior to systematic biopsy (positive biopsy rates 10.4% vs 5.3%, respectively).[63] Other studies have confirmed that CEUS improves cancer detection,[64] although no advantage of power or color Doppler has been shown.

Aigner and colleagues[65] compared CEUS-targeted biopsies with 10 core systematic biopsies in 44 patients. CEUS-targeted biopsies were positive in 105/220 biopsies (47%) with false positives in 20% of patients compared with positive biopsies in 41/440 (9%) systematic biopsies. There was no difference in Gleason score. Mitterberger and colleagues[66] studied 690 patients, comparing CEUS-targeted biopsies with systematic biopsies, and found higher Gleason scores in the targeted group (Gleason score 6.8 vs 5.4 [$P<.003$]).

Sedelaar and colleagues[67] showed a correlation between microvessel density and three-dimensional contrast-enhanced power Doppler imaging. Unal and colleagues[68] showed that contrast-enhanced power Doppler could be used to discriminate between benign prostatic hyperplasia and cancer with an accuracy of 81%.

Enhanced Doppler has also been used to monitor response to treatment. In a study of 68

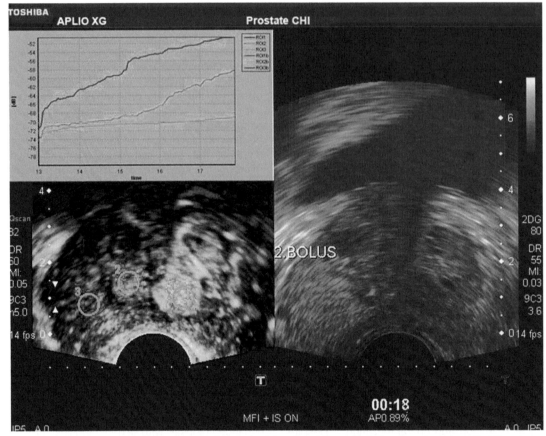

Fig. 19. Transverse image of the prostate imaged with a low-MI mode (Microflow Imaging, Toshiba, Japan) showing ROIs drawn on 3 areas in the prostate with their TICs above. (*Courtesy of* Professor, Thomas AC Fischer, Charite Hospital, Berlin, Germany.)

patients followed up during treatment with enhanced power Doppler, most showed a decrease in vascularity within a day or so following commencement of antiandrogen therapy, which paralleled declining prostate-specific antigen (PSA) levels (**Fig. 21**).[69] In 2 cases, there was a discrepancy in that the vascularity remained high despite a decrease in PSA. These

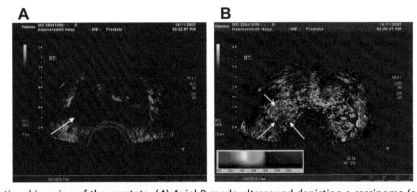

Fig. 20. Functional imaging of the prostate. (*A*) Axial B mode ultrasound depicting a carcinoma (*arrow*). (*B*) Corresponding section of prostate with a functional overlay image (Toshiba, Japan) superimposed showing contrast media bolus arrival time following an intravenous injection of microbubbles. The cancer (*arrows*) shows an earlier arrival time compared with the rest of the prostate. The color scale shows the arrival time in seconds. (*Reproduced from* Padhani AR, Harvey CJ, Cosgrove DO. Angiogenesis imaging in the management of prostate cancer. Nat Clin Pract Urol 2005;12:598; with permission.)

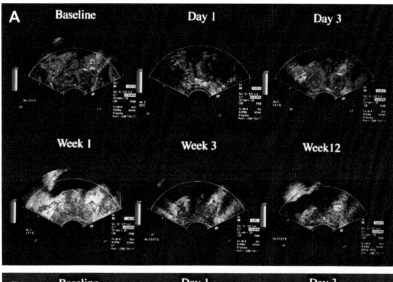

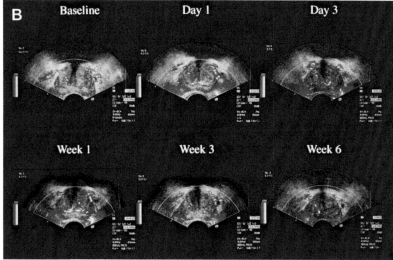

Fig. 21. Two cases of carcinoma of the prostate showing differential response to antiandrogen therapy on CEUS. (*A*) Sequence of contrast-enhanced power Doppler images taken from the peak in enhancement at baseline and intervals after commencement of therapy. Note the marked decrease in signals after the first week, indicating good response to therapy, which was observed clinically. (*B*) Sequence of contrast-enhanced power Doppler images of a different patient taken from the peak in enhancement at baseline and intervals after commencement of therapy. Note that, in this case, the signals do not decrease in the treatment period. This patient escaped from hormonal control at 6-month review. (*Courtesy of* Dr R Eckersley, Department of Imaging, Hammersmith Hospital; *Reproduced from* Padhani AR, Harvey CJ, Cosgrove DO. Angiogenesis imaging in the management of prostate cancer. Nat Clin Pract Urol 2005;12:603; with permission.)

patients had escaped from hormonal control at 6-month review. Failure to switch off neovascularity may be an early indicator of relapse that could prompt a treatment adjustment. The emergence of angiogenesis inhibitors is also interesting, and enhanced US could provide a quantitative tool to monitor these agents.

Targeted microbubbles are being developed that bind to specific markers or tissues and would greatly improve sensitivity.

Currently, the results of large multicentre trials are awaited comparing targeted postcontrast biopsies with systematic biopsies to ascertain whether the promise of CEUS of the prostate can be translated into clinical practice.

Ultrasound Microbubble Drug and Gene Delivery

Microbubbles can be used a vehicles to transport and deliver genes and drugs to a designated organ or target site such as a thrombus, in the case of thrombolytics, or a tumor. Delivery to a target site can be accentuated by incorporating ligands onto the microbubble that recognize receptors on the cell membrane.

US has been shown to cause a transient increase in cell membrane permeability in a process known as sonoporation. Using this technique, tissues can be targeted so that cellular uptake of a drug (eg, a chemotherapeutic agent) or gene is achieved.[70] Sonoporation requires high acoustic power (beyond that used in the diagnostic range but equivalent to those used in physiotherapy), but the power needed is markedly reduced when microbubbles are present. A drug or gene vector can be incorporated in or on the surface of the microbubbles, tracked in the circulation with an imaging beam, and, when they are exposed to high-power US, the microspheres rupture, releasing the agent in the vicinity of the target tissue.[71]

In oncological drugs, this has the advantage of decreasing the dose of the drug needed, thereby reducing systemic side effects. Encouraging initial in vitro studies have shown cell membrane sonoporation without inducing cell death. Animal work has been encouraging[72–74] but no human trials have been performed.

Limitations

There are some limitations of CEUS in the kidneys. In general, if the lesion is difficult to see on B mode, it may also be hard to find on CEUS because there is some loss of spatial resolution inherent in the contrast-specific modes. In obese patients, lesions high under the left hemidiaphragm and deep-sited lesions (>10 cm), CEUS may be difficult to perform and interpret. Because of the high cortical perfusion, medullary lesions may be obscured, especially if a 2.4-mL dose of SonoVue is given. A lower 1-mL dose is recommended to avoid this problem. In addition, simultaneous comparison with the contralateral kidney is not possible as with CT, MR, and intravenous urography. UCAs cannot provide information about the excretory function of the kidneys because these agents are purely intravascular.

SUMMARY

CEUS is a repeatable, real-time, multiplanar imaging modality that uses the only completely intravascular contrast agent in radiological imaging. CEUS is noninvasive, with no radiation exposure, may be used in renal impairment, obstruction, and in patients with contraindications for the use of contrast agents in CT or MR imaging.

CEUS can characterize indeterminate renal lesions, complex cysts, and focal inflammatory lesions. Contrast-enhanced ultrasound is excellent for assessing the renal vasculature and can be used in the diagnosis of renal artery stenosis, renal infarction, renal arterial/venous thrombosis, trauma, as well as the quantification of cortical perfusion. CEUS is a valuable addition to the Radiologist's armory, enabling increased confidence in the diagnosis and characterization of renal disorders to rival CT and MR imaging.

REFERENCES

1. Claudon M, Cosgrove D, Albrecht T, et al. Guidelines and good clinical practice recommendations for contrast enhanced ultrasound (CEUS) - update 2008. Ultraschall Med 2008;29:28–44.
2. Harvey C, Albrecht T. Ultrasound of focal liver lesions. Eur Radiol 2001;11:1578–93.
3. Robbin M, Lockhart M, Barr R. Renal imaging with ultrasound contrast: current status. Radiol Clin North Am 2003;41:963–78.
4. Setola S, Catalano O, Sandomenico F, et al. Contrast-enhanced sonography of the kidney. Abdom Imaging 2007;32:21–8.
5. Correas JM, Claudon M, Tranquart F, et al. The kidney: imaging with microbubble contrast agents. Ultrasound Q 2006;22:53–66.
6. Piscaglia F, Bolondi L. The safety of SonoVue in abdominal applications: retrospective analysis of 23188 investigations. Ultrasound Med Biol 2006;32:1369–75.
7. Quaia E. Microbubble ultrasound contrast agents: an update. Eur Radiol 2007;17:1995–2008.
8. Harvey CJ, Blomley MJ, Eckersley RJ, et al. Developments in ultrasound contrast media. Eur Radiol 2001;11:675–89.
9. Cosgrove D, Harvey C. Clinical uses of microbubbles in diagnosis and treatment. Med Biol Eng Comput 2009;47:813–26.
10. Cosgrove DO, Eckersley RJ, Blomley M, et al. Quantification of blood flow. Eur Radiol 2001;11:1338–44.
11. Wei K, Jayaweera AR, Firoozan S, et al. Quantification of myocardial blood flow with ultrasound induced destruction of microbubbles administered as a constant venous infusion. Circulation 1998;97:473–83.
12. Lassau N, Koscielny S, Albiges L, et al. Metastatic renal cell carcinoma treated with sunitinib: early evaluation of treatment response using dynamic contrast-enhanced ultrasonography. Clin Cancer Res 2010;16:1216–25.
13. Yeh HC, Halton KP, Shapiro RS, et al. Junctional parenchyma: revised definition of hypertrophic column of Bertin. Radiology 1992;185:725–32.

14. Bhatt S, MacLennan G, Dogra V. Renal pseudotumors. Am J Roentgenol 2007;188:1380–7.
15. Ascenti G, Zimbaro G, Mazziotti S, et al. Contrast-enhanced power Doppler US in the diagnosis of renal pseudotumours. Eur Radiol 2001;11:2496–9.
16. Israel GM, Bosniak MA. An update of the Bosniak renal cyst classification system. Urology 2005;66:484–8.
17. Ascenti G, Mazziotti S, Zimbaro G, et al. Complex cystic renal masses: characterization with contrast-enhanced US. Radiology 2007;243:158–65.
18. Park BK, Kim B, Kim SH, et al. Assessment of cystic renal masses based on Bosniak classification: comparison of CT and contrast-enhanced US. Eur J Radiol 2007;61:310–4.
19. Quaia E, Bertolotto M, Cioffi V, et al. Comparison of contrast-enhanced sonography with unenhanced sonography and contrast-enhanced ct in the diagnosis of malignancy in complex cystic renal masses. Am J Roentgenol 2008;191:1239–49.
20. Jamis-Dow CA, Choyke PL, Jennings SB, et al. Small (< or = 3cm) renal masses: detection with CT versus US and pathologic correlation. Radiology 1996;198:785–8.
21. Tamai H, Takiguchi Y, Oka M, et al. Contrast-enhanced ultrasonography in the diagnosis of solid renal tumors. J Ultrasound Med 2005;24:1635–40.
22. Leveridge MJ, Bostrom PJ, Koulouris G, et al. Imaging renal cell carcinoma with ultrasonography, CT and MRI. Nat Rev Urol 2010;7:311–25.
23. Quaia E, Siracusano S, Bertolotto M, et al. Characterization of renal tumours with pulse inversion harmonic imaging by intermittent high mechanical index technique: initial results. Eur Radiol 2003;13:1402–12.
24. Rioja J, de la Rosette JJ, Wijkstra H, et al. Advances in diagnosis and follow-up in kidney cancer. Curr Opin Urol 2008;18:447–54.
25. Xu ZF, Xu HX, Xie XY, et al. Renal cell carcinoma and renal angiomyolipoma: Differential diagnosis with real-time contrast enhanced ultrasonography. J Ultrasound Med 2010;29:709–17.
26. Ascenti G, Zimbaro G, Mazziotti S, et al. Usefulness of power Doppler and contrast-enhanced sonography in the differentiation of hyperechoic renal masses. Abdom Imaging 2001;26:654–60.
27. Ascenti G, Gaeta M, Magno C, et al. Contrast-enhanced second-harmonic sonography in the detection of pseudocapsule in renal cell carcinoma. AJR Am J Roentgenol 2004;182:1525–30.
28. Meister M, Choyke P, Anderson C, et al. Radiological evaluation, management, and surveillance of renal masses in Von Hippel-Lindau disease. Clin Radiol 2009;64:589–600.
29. Ogan K, Jacomides L, Dolmatch BL, et al. Percutaneous radiofrequency ablation of renal tumors: technique, limitations, and morbidity. Urology 2002;60:954–8.
30. Tracy CR, Raman JD, Donnally C, et al. Durable oncologic outcomes after radiofrequency ablation: experience from treating 243 small renal masses over 7.5 years. Cancer 2010;116:3135–42.
31. Kim JH, Eun HW, Lee HK, et al. Renal perfusion abnormality. Coded harmonic angio US with contrast agent. Acta Radiol 2003;44:166–71.
32. Claudon M, Plouin PF, Baxter GM, et al. Renal arteries in patients at risk of renal artery stenosis: multicenter evaluation of the echo-enhancer SHU 508A at color and spectral Doppler US. Levovist Renal Artery Stenosis Group. Radiology 2000;214:739–46.
33. Sidhu R, Lockhart ME. Imaging of renovascular disease. Semin Ultrasound CT MR 2009;30:271–88.
34. Wei K, Le E, Bin JP, et al. Quantification of renal blood-flow with contrast-enhanced ultrasound. J Am Coll Cardiol 2001;37:1135–40.
35. Owen DR, Shalhoub J, Miller S, et al. Inflammation within carotid atherosclerotic plaque: assessment with late-phase contrast-enhanced US. Radiology 2010;255:638–44.
36. Lavocat M, Granjou D, Allard D, et al. Imaging of pyelonephritis. Pediatr Radiol 1997;27:159–65.
37. Farhat W, Traubici J, Sherman C, et al. Reliability of contrast enhanced sonography with harmonic imaging for detecting early renal scarring in experimental pyelonephritis in a porcine model: preliminary results. J Urol 2002;168:1114–7.
38. Kim B, Lim HK, Choi MH, et al. Detection of parenchymal abnormalities in acute pyelonephritis by pulse inversion harmonic imaging with or without microbubble ultrasonographic contrast agent: correlation with computed tomography. J Ultrasound Med 2001;20:5–14.
39. Mitterberger M, Pinggera G, Colleselli D, et al. Acute pyelonephritis: comparison of diagnosis with computed tomography and contrast-enhanced ultrasonography. BJU Int 2008;101:341–4.
40. Catalano O, Aiani L, Barozzi L, et al. CEUS in abdominal trauma: multi-center study. Abdom Imaging 2009;34:225–34.
41. Valentino M, Ansaloni L, Catena F, et al. Contrast-enhanced ultrasonography in blunt abdominal trauma: considerations after 5 years of experience. Radiol Med 2009;114:1080–93.
42. Kay DH, Mazonakis M, Geddes C, et al. Ultrasonic microbubble contrast agents and the transplant kidney. Clin Radiol 2009;64:1081–7.
43. Kihm LP, Hinkel UP, Michael K, et al. Contrast-enhanced sonography shows superior microvascular renal allograft perfusion in patients switched from cyclosporine A to everolimus. Transplantation 2009;88:261–5.
44. Lebkowska U, Janica J, Lebkowski W, et al. Renal parenchyma perfusion spectrum and resistive index

(RI) in ultrasound examinations with contrast medium in the early period after kidney transplantation. Transplant Proc 2009;41:3024–7.

45. Jimenez C, Lopez MO, Gonzalez E, et al. Ultrasonography in kidney transplantation: values and new developments. Transplant Rev (Orlando) 2009;23:209–13.

46. Schwenger V, Korosoglou G, Hinkel UP, et al. Real-time contrast-enhanced sonography of renal transplant recipients predicts chronic allograft nephropathy. Am J Transplant 2006;6:609–15.

47. Darge K, Zieger B, Rohrschneider W, et al. Contrast-enhanced harmonic imaging for the diagnosis of vesicoureteric reflux in pediatric patients. AJR Am J Roentgenol 2001;177:1411–5.

48. Ascenti G, Zimbaro G, Mazziotti S, et al. Harmonic US imaging of vesicoureteric reflux in children: usefulness of a second generation contrast agent. Pediatr Radiol 2004;34:481–7.

49. Darge K. Voiding urosonography with US contrast agent for the diagnosis of vesicoureteric reflux in children: an update. Pediatr Radiol 2010;40:956–62.

50. Papadopoulou F, Anthopoulou A, Siomou E, et al. Harmonic voiding urosonography with a second-generation contrast agent for the diagnosis of vesicoureteral reflux. Pediatr Radiol 2009;39: 239–44.

51. Darge K, Beer M, Gordjani N, et al. Contrast-enhanced voiding urosonography with the use of a 2nd generation US contrast medium: preliminary result. Pediatr Radiol 2004;34:S31.

52. Darge K. Voiding urosonography with ultrasound contrast agents for the diagnosis of vesicoureteric reflux in children. Pediatr Radiol 2008;38:40–63.

53. Bigler SA, Deering RE, Brawer MK. Comparison of microscopic vascularity in benign and malignant prostate tissue. Hum Pathol 1993;24:220–6.

54. Padhani AR, Harvey CJ, Cosgrove DO. Angiogenesis imaging in the management of prostate cancer. Nat Clin Pract Urol 2005;12:596–607.

55. Ferrara K, Merritt C, Burns P, et al. Evaluation of tumour angiogenesis with US: imaging, Doppler and contrast agents. Acad Radiol 2000;7:824–39.

56. Harvey CJ, Pilcher J, Eckersley R, et al. Advances in ultrasound. Clin Radiol 2002;57:157–77.

57. Eckersley RJ, Cosgrove DO, Blomley MJ, et al. Functional imaging of tissue response to bolus injection of ultrasound contrast agent. Proc IEEE Ultrason Symp 1998;2:1779–82.

58. Grossen TE, Sedelaar JP, De la Rosette JJ, et al. The value of dynamic contrast enhanced power Doppler ultrasound in the localization of prostatic carcinoma [abstract 355]. Eur Urol 2002;1:91.

59. Rickards D, Gillams AR, Deng J, et al. Do intravascular ultrasound Doppler contrast agents improve transrectal ultrasound diagnosis of prostate cancer. Radiology 1998;209:182.

60. Halpern EJ, Rosenberg M, Gomella LG. Prostate cancer: contrast enhanced US for detection. Radiology 2001;219:219–25.

61. Frauscher F, Klauser A, Halpern EJ. Advances in ultrasound for the detection of prostate cancer. Ultrasound Q 2002;18:135–42.

62. Frauscher F, Klauser A, Halpern EJ. Detection of prostate cancer with a microbubble contrast agent. Lancet 2001;357:1849–50.

63. Frauscher F, Klauser A, Volgger H, et al. Comparison of contrast-enhanced color Doppler targeted biopsy with conventional systematic biopsy: impact on prostate cancer. J Urol 2002;167:1648–52.

64. Halpern EJ, Frauscher F, Rosenberg M, et al. Directed biopsy during contrast enhanced sonography of the prostate. AJR Am J Roentgenol 2002; 178:915–9.

65. Aigner F, Pallwein L, Mitterberger M, et al. Contrast-enhanced ultrasonography using cadence-contrast pulse sequencing technology for targeted biopsy of the prostate. BJU Int 2009;103:458–63.

66. Mitterberger M, Pinggera GM, Horninger W, et al. Comparison of contrast enhanced color Doppler targeted biopsy to conventional systematic biopsy: impact on Gleason score. J Urol 2007;178:464–8.

67. Sedelaar JP, Van Leenders GJ, Hulsbergen-Van De Kaa CA, et al. Microvessel density: correlation between contrast ultrasonography and histology of prostate cancer. Eur Urol 2001;40:285–93.

68. Unal D, Sedelaar JP, Aarnink RG, et al. Three-dimensional contrast-enhanced power Doppler ultrasonography and conventional examination methods: the value of diagnostic predictors of prostate cancer. BJU Int 2000;86:58–64.

69. Eckersley RJ, Butler-Barnes J, Blomley MJ, et al. Quantification microbubble enhanced transrectal ultrasound (TRUS) as a tool for monitoring anti-androgen therapy in prostate carcinoma. Radiology 1998;209:310.

70. Liang HD, Tang J, Halliwell M. Sonoporation, drug delivery, and gene therapy. Proc Inst Mech Eng H 2010;224:343–61.

71. Unger EC. Targeting and delivery of drugs with contrast agents. In: Thomsen HS, Muller RN, Mattrey RF, editors. Trends in contrast media. Medical radiology: diagnostic imaging and radiation oncology series. Berlin (Germany): Springer; 1999. p. 405–12.

72. Koike H, Tomita N, Azuma H, et al. An efficient gene transfer method mediated by ultrasound and microbubbles into the kidney. J Gene Med 2005;7:108–16.

73. van der Wouden EA, Sandovici M, Henning RH, et al. Approaches and methods in gene therapy for kidney disease. J Pharmacol Toxicol Methods 2004;50:13–24.

74. Isaka Y. Gene therapy targeting kidney diseases: routes and vehicles. Clin Exp Nephrol 2006;10: 229–35.

Index

Printed and bound by CPI Group (UK) Ltd, Croydon, CR0 4YY

03/10/2024

01040351-0015